Our Synthetic Environment

Our Synthetic Environment

REVISED EDITION

MURRAY BOOKCHIN

HARPER COLOPHON BOOKS
Harper & Row, Publishers
New York, Evanston, San Francisco, London

This book was originally published in a hardcover edition by Alfred A. Knopf in 1962.

First HARPER COLOPHON edition published 1974

STANDARD BOOK NUMBER: 06–090363–5

To Rose, my mother

(1895–1961)

ACKNOWLEDGMENTS

THE BASIC VIEWS presented in this book were nourished by many sources. My opinions on problems of human biology and health have been influenced primarily by the work of the great Nobel laureate Alexis Carrel; those on agriculture and ecology are based in large part on the writings of Professors William A. Albrecht and Charles Elton. I profited immensely from Professor Hans Selye's works on stress and from Lewis Mumford's studies on urban development.

I wish to extend my gratitude to a grand lady and gallant conservationist, Dr. Margaret Nice, for reading the portion of my book on pesticides and wildlife, and to thank Lewis Mumford for reading my discussion of urban life. I benefited a great deal from the suggestions of Dr. Joseph Meiers, who read my discussion of stress and enriched it with his extensive professional background in neuropsychiatry. I am grateful to Alex Scher for reading Chapter Four and answering many questions on food technology; to Professor Francis E. Ray, director of the Cancer Research Laboratory, University of Florida, for reading and offering valuable advice on Chapter Five; to Professors Jack Schwartz, Mathematics Institute, New York University, John M. Fowler, Physics Department, Washington University, and Barry Commoner, Committee on Molecular Biology, Washington University, for reading and making useful suggestions on Chapter Six. I am especially indebted to F. J. Schlink, technical director of Consumers' Research and editor of *Consumer Bulletin,* for reading and offering many suggestions on portions of my book on food additives and food and drug control. I regret that limitations of space made it impossible for me to provide the reader with the wealth of material that Consumers' Research has accumulated on these problems. I am grateful to many research workers in agronomy, radiobiology, medicine, and public health who responded to my requests for opinions, data, and in some cases, unpublished works. Although I owe much to the work and generosity of others, I wish to claim full responsibility for the views presented in this book.

The original version of this book could not have been written without the encouragement and editorial assistance of my former wife, Beatrice Bookchin, my editor, Angus Cameron, and my friends David Eisen, Mrs. Beverly Fetterman, and Burton Lasky. For help in preparing the Colophon Edition, I would like to express my deep appreciation to the two fine editors, Hugh Van Dusen and Cynthia Merman, whose suggestions contributed to the current version of the book. Finally I am profoundly indebted to my close friends and colleagues at the Center for New Studies at Mahwah, New Jersey, notably Gina Blumenfeld, Emily Boardman, Trent Schroyer, and Joel Whitebook, who have been continuing sources of insight and personal support.

CONTENTS

INTRODUCTION TO THE
COLOPHON EDITION

ALTHOUGH MORE than twelve years has passed since *Our Synthetic Environment* was first published, the book seems as contemporary and relevant today as it did in the early sixties. On rereading it, I find very little I would want to change. The environmental deterioration, which the book emphasized and documented so painstakingly, has worsened since 1962 and perhaps taken more sinister forms. We are confronted as seriously with the problems of subclinical illness, the changing spectrum of disease, soil deterioration, low-quality food, urban breakdown, chemical food additives, environmental cancer from air, water and radioactive pollution—in short, the grave problems of "human ecology"—as we were more than a decade ago. Our major concern for radioactive pollution may center less on surface bomb tests than on the "peacetime" uses of nuclear energy, and the United States has greatly diminished its use of DDT—which is not to say that even these specific problems have disappeared, as witness French and Chinese surface tests, venting of radioactive material from underground explosions by the United States and Russia, and the growing use of DDT as part of the "green revolution" abroad. What gives significance to *Our Synthetic Environment* are the underlying principles of social ecology and public health that the data were meant to support. As the fine biologist William Vogt observed in a review of the book, I was concerned not with a factual muckraking of episodic abuses, but with humanity's most fundamental relationships with the natural world. The data, however significant and revealing in themselves, were meant to illustrate the grave crisis that was emerging from modern society's attempt to "dominate" nature.

To readers of the seventies who have experienced "Earth Day" and an overly rhetorical social commitment to ecological values, it is very difficult to convey the prejudices this message encountered twelve years ago. *Our Synthetic Environment* was published under my penname of "Lewis Herber" by Alfred A. Knopf, Inc., in the spring of 1962, roughly a half-year before Rachel Carson's *Silent Spring* appeared in book form. Despite the encouragement of a prestigious publisher and an outstanding editor, it stood almost alone in its vulnerability to the biases of the time. The controversy that exploded around Rachel Carson's book in the autumn of the same year, a book by a poetic nature writer who enjoys an almost reverential following by millions of readers, highlights the extent to which American public opinion, orchestrated by corporate interests and governmental agencies, adhered to a "grow or die" economic mentality and a domineering attitude toward the natural world. The prevailing attitude of that time is perhaps best illustrated by a *New York Times* review of the book that opined that, while *Our Synthetic Environment* "tackles the full range of the [environmental] problem" and "does sound the alarm," its sentiments were "nice" but "impossible."[1] The book, in fact, was patronized to death by a flippant commitment to the status quo— in effect, to an increasingly chemicalized agriculture, more pesticides and food additives, larger nuclear plants, and ever-greater urbanization. "Mistakes will be made that cannot be corrected," concluded the critic, "but only deplored in retrospect, for man is human after all. The best we can hope for is that he will be sufficiently aware of the risk to guard intelligently against repeating past error or making new ones." So much for the "best we can hope for." By dint of sheer misreading, "Mr. Herber" was treated as atavistic: "No one is going to stop the world so that some who would like to get off will be able to or, as with Mr. Herber, spin us backward in time."[2] These words should not be dismissed as fatuous platitudes. The critic, a fairly prominent *New York Times* reporter, essentially echoed a sentiment that was characteristic of the country as a whole—the equating of "progress" with mindless growth and the technocratic ideal of "progress above all." To suggest that pesticides, food additives, chemicalized agriculture, burgeoning urbanization, and nuclear energy were harmful was regarded not merely as "reactionary" but as a national heresy.

And with heresy went the most shameless mobilization of propaganda and punitive action the country had seen since the McCarthy period a decade earlier. The food, chemical, agricultural, and pharmaceutical industries seemed to unite with the American Medical Association, the Department of Agriculture, the Atomic Energy Commission, and the Food and Drug Administration to launch a massive program of "informing" the public on the advantages it gained from pesticides, chemicals in food, and nuclear power plants, while, more quietly, court suits and injunctions faced "crackpots" who dared to question seriously the spirit of "progress" that percolated through the land. For an agronomist to suggest that there was any virtue in organic farming, for a physician to imply that conventional medicine did not provide the ultimate in therapy, for an urbanologist to urge the decentralization of the cities, for an ecologist to stress that chemistry did not afford the exclusive bridge between humanity and nature, and quite generally, for anyone to denounce the promises afforded by nuclear power was to risk more than professional denunciation. Such individuals were often ostracized, if not characterized as "quacks," and in some cases actually jailed. The *Times* critic of *Our Synthetic Environment*, in fact, was quite mild. His criticism had appeared in the paper fully a year after the book had been published, when attacks on envionmentalists had already been tempered by Rachel Carson's *Silent Spring*. It was reviewed not as a a precursor of Carson's admirable work but as one of many books that had followed in its tow.

Our Synthetic Environment, however, also had its supporters—not only in Vogt and in a number of courageous newspaper reviewers, but also in René Dubos, that grand old man of social ecology who added his own considerable professional background and literary skill to the cause of environmental improvement. Dubos brought the book to the attention of his colleagues in professional journals and in his own volumes. Generally, the book found its best reception among the technically trained rather than the general public, which understandably was captivated by the superb prose of *Silent Spring*. Having sold out fairly rapidly, *Our Synthetic Environment* became a widely bibliographed but not easily obtainable work and tended to attract the sophisticated connoisseur of environmental issues rather than the exuberant activist.

Today, we have all become sophisticated in environmental issues, and the book can be expected to enjoy a much wider readership than it had in 1962. It is no longer necessary to define the word "ecology"; everyone, presumably, knows what the word means, and it drops from the lips as readily and piously as the word "motherhood." Indeed, it is used a little too uncritically—to a point where "ecology" and "environmentalism" have become interchangeable terms. Ecology, in my view, refers to a broad, philosophical, almost spiritual, outlook toward humanity's relationship to the natural world, not merely to a scientific discipline or pragmatic technique. "Environmentalism," by contrast, is a form of natural engineering that seeks to manipulate nature as mere "natural resources" with minimal pollution and public outcry. Environmentalists, such as Mr. Nixon, are not ecologists, nor do I regard serious ecologists as environmentalists.

Our Synthetic Environment is unique in more respects than its broad scope and its anticipation of issues that were to become rooted in public consciousness during the late sixties. It went further than *Silent Spring*, a work which focused almost entirely on pesticides. This heterodoxy and range give it striking relevance to our own times, particularly when one examines the specific issues it raises. The term "subclinical" (or latent) disease, for example, did not enjoy great popularity in the medical community of the early sixties. Medicine and the life sciences generally had become almost physical sciences. Researchers were deeply enamored of biochemistry, quantitative studies, and overt symptoms that could be clearly measured and recorded. To argue that cancer developed slowly in the body over various precancerous stages; to claim that it was a systemic condition based on the overall health of the individual, not simply a local one that could be viewed as the misbehavior of cells, tissues, or a specific organ; to hope for its cure in a better understanding of the body's immunological mechanisms, not merely in radiation and chemical therapy—all of these arguments, so exciting and prominent today, were not acknowledged readily by the profession a dozen years ago. True, arguments of this kind had been advanced much earlier by lonely figures such as Sigismund Peller, at Johns Hopkins and New York University medical schools, but they were unknown even to fairly well informed general readers and, indeed, to many professional people. Peller's work *Cancer in Man* was justly described as "a fighting book."[3] Only in recent years has the profession been willing to deal seriously with such arguments and to pursue them vigorously as research projects.

The book's view of soil as a "palpitating sheet of life," while I attributed it to agronomy as a whole, actually involved a radical cleavage with the prevailing views of American agricultural schools at the time. Its prudent endorsement of organic farming, its respect for every plot of land "as a small, highly individuated cosmos," its emphasis on the relationship between soil fertility and the quality of foods, and its attack upon agribusiness were regarded as rank heresy—almost the object of juridical retribution. If courses in organic agriculture are now part of the curricula of many American agricultural colleges, it is difficult to convey the savage hostility any sympathetic treatment of the subject evoked in the early sixties among conventional agronomists, the food industry, the Food and Drug Administration, and even the American Medical Association. A sizable article I had written on this subject as early as 1952 in the Anglo-

American quarterly *Contemporary Issues* went largely unnoticed in the United States—so far removed was the issue from public interest—although it aroused considerable attention in Germany, where it was published in several editions as a paperback book. The situation was even more embattled ten years later when *Our Synthetic Environment* appeared. To impute any significance to organic farming might easily have involved a legal battle with the Food and Drug Administration. Here, too, I must add a word of tribute to a gallant man, William A. Albrecht, Professor Emeritus of Soils at the University of Missouri, who almost alone withstood the professional pressures of the period and wrote the original introduction to *Our Synthetic Environment*.

The book is unique also in terms of the synergistic activity—the more-than-additive effect—it imputes to chemicals in food and other pollutants. Today it is difficult to believe that carbon monoxide was not regarded as a serious air pollutant twelve years ago. It was only by means of painstaking effort that I could acquire authoritative opinions that regarded the gas as a serious environmental danger. The literature of the late fifties stressed the transient nature of carbon monoxide and its insignificance as an air pollutant. Moreover, the literature took no notice of the effect carbon monoxide from motor vehicles and cigarettes, combined with nitrites in processed meat, had on the oxygen-carrying capacity of the blood. The issue of synergistic effects and the combined effect of carbon monoxide and nitrites on people with heart disease is now an important issue in environmental studies. Here, too, *Our Synthetic Environment* could justly claim to have been far in advance of its time. Its data on this score are as applicable today as they were a dozen years ago—and certainly more readily acknowledged as issues requiring careful study.

I could easily adduce many such examples that anticipate problems and issues that are coming into focus during the 1970s. To my mind it is most important to stress the larger ecological framework that these examples try to support and the radical solutions that the book proposes in its concluding pages. *Our Synthetic Environment*, although giving due acknowledgment to the need for arresting environmental breakdown in every way possible, does not stop with mere reforms. The book's critique is directed at the social order as a whole. It demands a radical decentralization of the cities, new systems of energy and food cultivation, and a rational ecological society. In advancing this viewpoint, the book also divorces itself from the shallow notions of human ecology that were current at the time. The popular concept of a "magic bullet"—of a single recipe—that would cope with all our physical problems is replaced by a totalistic view of health. Indeed, the emphasis in *Our Synthetic Environment* is on promoting health rather than curing disease. And just as the book rejects chemical therapy as an exclusive means for dealing with illness, so too it rejects all one-sided panaceas, such as exotic foods, vitamins, organic fertilizers, or special exercises. Health is seen as emerging from a healthy way of life, not from any single element that might enter into making such a way of life. Only a rounded and healthful environment that includes a sound diet of good foods, physical as well as intellectual activity, spiritual insight as well as unpolluted air and water—all of these and more—will yield a rounded and healthy human being. Ultimately, such a rounded and healthy environment presupposes the existence of a rounded and healthy society. Accordingly, *Our Synthetic Environment* is concerned not only with the relationship of humanity to nature and the balance of nature; it is even more fundamentally con-

cerned with the relationship between human and human.
The book advances the notion that there can be no sound
natural environment without a sound, ecologically oriented social environment.

I have already noted that, despite the passing of
twelve years, there is little I would remove from *Our
Synthetic Environment*. A year or two years ago I might
have conceded that pages dealing with DDT, certain
cancer-causing food additives, and the increase in radioactive isotopes in the human food chain required alteration.
Not that any of the broader problems have disappeared;
but in certain specific details, I had hoped that they
would require less emphasis than they received in
the original version of the book. Now I must confess that
the details of my discussion in these pages are also as
relevant as they were a dozen years ago. An ongoing
assault has been mounted by agribusiness and the food
industry, with considerable administration support,
against the 1958 Delaney "anticancer clause" in the Food,
Drug and Cosmetic Act. The open hostility of Robert
Finch, Mr. Nixon's more "liberal" HEW secretary, to the
Delaney clause during the famous "cyclamate crisis" of
1970 (about which more later) has, in my opinion,
merely placed the Food and Drug Administration's opposition to the amendment behind the closed doors of the
agency's upper echelons since Mr. Finch's departure.
That the amendment will be challenged repeatedly in the
future as "unrealistic"—if not juridically, then in the
day-to-day practices of the food industry and the FDA—is
a certainty. Attempts are clearly being made at this writing to restore the use of banned, almost grotesquely
harmful agents such as the synthetic estrogen diethylstilbestrol (DES) and even DDT, despite pious commit-
ments to keep these potent toxicants and carcinogens out

of the American diet. The decision by U.S. Court of Appeals Judge Harold Leventhal in January 1974, to lift the DES ban because the FDA failed to follow "sound administrative procedure" and used what the court described as "scare tactics "is one of many typical setbacks that face the American public. That the FDA's "administrative procedure" left the agency open to this decision raises the question not only of the court's biased verbiage ("scare tactics") and the interests this language serves but also the FDA's curious behavior in rendering the DES ban so vulnerable to a judicial upset.

It requires no scare tactics to feel very uncomfortable about DES, or "stilbestrol," as it is called in this book. My account of its hazards is as valid today as when it was first written. Banned years ago for use in poultry destined for interstate sale (although it was extensively used in intrastate sales), DES remained an integral part of cattle fattening procedures in feedlots up to 1973 when researchers, using highly sophisticated analytic techniques, found residues in the parts per billion in cattle livers sold to the public. The most minute residues of this synthetic estrogen must be viewed with the greatest suspicion. Given variations in individual responses, the quantitative impact of hormonal agents like DES is utterly unpredictable. Such agents have been likened to sprinklings of dynamite on a roaring fire: they may crackle and disappear—or explode. Yet even an environmentally oriented newspaper like *The New York Times* editorially opined last year that the FDA's banning of DES in such minute residues was extravagant. If this is the opinion of the *Times*, one may well imagine the opinion of business and the administration.

The pious vows by public officials at all levels of government to avoid the use of DDT are now giving way to disgruntled demands for once again employing this highly dangerous pesticide. State forestry officials in the Northwest have joined private lumber interests in exerting pressure on the federal Environmental Protection Agency for relaxing the nation-wide DDT ban to control the Douglas Fir Tussock moth. Currently, some state officials have indicated they might have recourse to legal action against the EPA. The demands and threats come at a time when research indicates that DDT may interfere with the reproduction of mammals as well as birds by lengthening the oestrus cycle and lowering the frequency with which fertilized ova develop. Indeed, a recent independent study of California sea lions suggests that high DDT levels in the diet, which appear in the fat depots of these animals, causes premature births.

In any case, the widely touted ban on DDT has not diminished human and animal exposure to the group of highly dangerous chlorinated hydrocarbons in which the pesticide is classified. Aldrin and dieldrin, both chlorinated hydrocarbon pesticides, are still widely used in American agriculture despite their close similarity, chemically and in terms of their physiological activity, to DDT. Dieldrin, the pesticide into which aldrin decomposes, has been found in suckling infants at levels thirty times the maximum permissible amount designated by the World Health Organization. Efforts by the EPA to ban these pesticides have met with stiff legal resistance from industry and, characteristically, from the U.S. Department of Agriculture.*

Short of banning or placing very severe restrictions on the use of chlorinated hydrocarbons, there is very little likelihood that this highly toxic spectrum of compounds can be kept out of the human food chain. We were scarcely alerted to the hazards of DDT, DDE, aldrin,

* Aldrin and dieldrin were finally banned by the EPA in August 1974.

dieldrin, chlordane, and other chlorinated pesticides when Swedish researchers in the mid-sixties began to report the presence of a seemingly new chlorinated hydrocarbon in the environment. I refer to the poly-chlorinated biphenyls (PCBs), a group of agents that are used as plasticizers, flame retardants, insulating fluids, and as mixers for enhancing the "kill-life" of chlorinated pesticides. The similarity of the PCBs to DDT is so close that initially the former were mistaken for the latter in environmental bioassays. Initially detected in fish and birds, the PCBs are now commonplace in human food. A recent FDA survey of some 3,500 samples of milk, cheese, eggs, and fish revealed that one out of five of these staples was measurably contaminated by the chlor-inated hydrocarbon, a substance which in the judgment of some researchers may be regarded as 100 times more toxic than DDT. Indeed, a recent evaluation of evidence by a federal researcher on the subject suggests that half of the world's human population may be carrying PCBs in its fat depots.

The physiological effects of PCBs could easily bog-gle the credulity of most individuals today. Michigan State University researchers found, for example, that episodes in which minks ceased to reproduce in ranches around the Great Lakes region were due to the presence of PCBs in Lake Michigan coho salmon fed to the ani-mals. Complete reproductive failure resulted from PCB levels of as little as five parts per million. PCBs produce the liver damage we associate with DDT. Also like DDT, the chlorinated hydrocarbon is stored in fat and is re-leased in appreciable quantities into the blood stream precisely when illness places the greatest physiological demands upon the body's fat reserves. Analyses of wild-life specimens reveal that PCBs are now ubiquitous. The Canadian Wildlife Service has found them in polar bears, seals, and fish thousands of miles from the nearest sites of industrial usage. As to the human food chain, the FDA's studies of commercial fish showed that 54 percent of the 670 specimens studied were contaminated by PCBs ranging from trace amounts to as much as 35 parts per million. Roughly 30 percent of the eggs analyzed by the FDA contained PCBs; nor is it any consolation to know that this percentage dropped in the case of cheese and milk to 6 and 7 percent respectively. One milk sample contained a PCB level as high as 30 parts per million.

Yet PCBs are not pesticides; they are not required to rescue a food crop from loss by pest infestations—to "feed the world" as agribusiness dramatically tries to remind us. They are industrial chemicals. Although they were first produced in 1929, their use on a wide scale is a comparatively recent phenomenon. Prior to the 1940s or 1950s, our high-technology civilization managed to produce plasticizers, sealants, printing inks, and heat-exchange fluids without using PCBs. The lavish use of these chlorinated hydrocarbons can be attributed more to the "chemo-mania" that enters into modern capitalism's value system of domination than to authentic social needs.

Metals and minerals, such as lead, mercury, asbestos, cadmium, and nickel, that I dealt with cursorily, if at all, and whose impact I necessarily disregarded for want of data in the early sixties, are now viewed as major air and water pollutants. Lead, almost militantly disregarded by FDA bureaucrats as a significant air pollutant, has been aptly described by Leonard Bruckman, senior air-pollution-control engineer in Connecticut's Department of Environmental Protection, as one of the most serious environmental poisons to which children are exposed. "In New Haven and Hartford, excessive lead exposures among children have reached epidemic proportions," Bruckman observes. "The mean outdoor lead content of Hartford street dirt is twice the Federal proposed maximum allowable level for lead in paint (0.06 percent). The fallout of lead from the air is a major contributor to the urban dirt lead content. . . . Nearly 95 percent of the total lead emitted into the Connecticut atmosphere is due to gasoline consumption. The potential adverse health effects caused by air lead fallout are chilling."[4]

These chilling effects should not go unmentioned. Lead, second only to iron as a metallic air pollutant, damages the liver, kidneys, central nervous system, brain, and reproductive system. Lead poisoning is marked by abdominal pains, vomiting, and with the progressive deterioration of the individual, paralysis, convulsions, and coma. Children are especially susceptible to the ingestion of lead; they may suffer not only damage to the nervous system, but mental retardation. Although the profession tends to deny the existence of sub-clinical damage from the metal, lead accumulates in bone, and for growing children, this cumulative effect may well shorten their life spans if rodent experiments with lead apply to humans. Leafy plants readily accumulate significant amounts of lead from motor vehicle exhausts; grass, growing near a secondary highway, was found to contain up to 200 parts per million. The subject of lead poisoning from gasoline exhausts had been virtually taboo for years by federal health officials, until independent studies indisputably established the metal as a major and very hazardous air pollutant, as ubiquitous in the environment as DDT, radioactive isotopes, and PCBs.

But the pollutant is not strictly derived from motor vehicle exhausts, although gasoline is by far its major source in the air. Aside from its presence in early paints, lead can also enter into food from antiquated canning techniques. During the summer of 1971, FDA researchers reported that lead in concentrations of 0.7 to 0.8 parts per million had been found in canned evaporated milk owing to the solder and flux used to seal the cans. Subsequent surveys have essentially confirmed these data. More recently, in May of last year, a New York State Health Department survey of canned fruit juice for babies revealed that 20 percent of 155 cans contained 0.4 parts per million or more of lead. Consumers Union, in a biting critique of FDA standards for lead in canned milk, observes that if one accepts the agency's "guideline maximum of 0.50 parts per million, a single 13-ounce can of evaporated milk is permitted to contain about 200 micrograms of lead, two-thirds of the child's maximum daily permissible intake from all sources." At which point, CU appropiately asks: "What, then, of the very young infant, who could well weigh only half as much as a one-year-old and who could easily consume a can of evaporated milk a day?"[5]

No less "chilling" are the effects of mercury, a pollutant that is now very widespread in water as well as air. Mercury poisoning can produce irreversible brain and neurological damage. A sizable proportion of people who are poisoned by the element die an agonizing death. Long regarded as a limited occupational hazard, mercury poisoning began to become a serious environmental issue in 1950 when Japanese fishermen in Minamata, a village on the shores of Yatsushiro Bay on Kyushu Island, began to notice inexplicably large fish kills. The fish, floating on the surface with strangely wide-open mouths, had died from mercury that entered the bay as effluent from the Chisso Corporation (then known as Nippon Nitrogen), an industrial installation on which more than two-thirds of the local economy depended. The mercury in the dead fish soon began to travel into the animal food chain: cats eating the discarded fish went into wild gyrations and died in agony. Pigs and dogs were described as "going mad"; birds that had apparently also consumed the dead fish dropped in mid-flight from the sky. In 1953 the pollutant claimed its first human victim in what became known as "Minamata disease," with its consequent brain damage, paralysis, loss of hearing and sight, and its effects on unborn children, a number of whom were born retarded or crippled. Before "Minamata disease" was checked, it had affected close to 400 people, of whom nearly 70 had died.

At this writing, the most comprehensive reviews of environmental mercury contamination appear, to the best of my knowledge, in the U.S. Interior Department's Geological Survey Professional Paper 713, "Mercury in the Environment." An estimated 23 million pounds of mercury are released worldwide into the environment each year. Mercury, to be sure, comes not only from industrial sources but also from natural ones, such as volcanic fumaroles, hot springs, tar pits, and oil field waters. In these cases, environmental contamination is unavoidable, although there is an obvious overlap between natural and industrial sources in the case of oil field waters. Intentional uses of mercury for industrial production results in considerable pollution. Of the 72,-000 metric tons mined and imported in the United States alone over the past forty years, "as much as 25 percent of this total may have been leaked into the environment," observes R. L. Wershaw in one of the Interior Department papers.[6] The widespread use of mercury compounds as fungicides, bacteriacides, and slimicides—in agriculture, regularly as a seed dressing—and their uses by the paint industry for mildew proofing, by the paper industry to prevent the growth of slimes in machinery, and by pharmaceutical and dental concerns, lead to public exposure on many different levels. Some papers are so high in mercury content that their use in food packaging is prohibited.

But perhaps even more serious is the "unintentional" mercury pollution from wastes that are the results of other industrial activities. "Minamata disease"—and the "disease" appeared in many areas other than communities around Yatshusiro Bay—resulted from mercury effluents that were released in the course of fairly commonplace petrochemical activities. According to recent data, coal-burning may be the largest single source of mercury in the environment. A typical 700 megawatt coal-burning plant often emits as much as 90 percent of the mercury present in the fuel. This is by no means a small quantity; a single plant alone has been found to emit 1,500 pounds of mercury annually in vaporized form. Averages of 1,000 pounds per year have been found in studies of eight Illinois power plants. The sensational tuna and swordfish episodes, which dramatically brought mercury pollution to widespread public attention in the United States, beggar these lesser known sources, such as power plants— sources that the "energy crisis," with its emphasis on a greater use of coal and its lower environmental standards, has further obscured.

An even more "'insidious threat to human health than mercury," observes Julian McCaull of *Environment* magazine, is the blue-tinged silvery element cadmium, which appears most commonly as a by-product of refining other metals but is also extensively used in industry.[7] The quantity of cadmium that appears in industrial products is more than double that of mercury. In Japan, cadmium poisoning from mining wastes resulted in hundreds of cases of severe degenerative bone disease. Twenty-five percent of the victims died. Many of the survivors suffered a grotesque crippling that left their limbs twisted and distorted. In the United States, a statistical survey of twenty-eight cities revealed a significant correlation of deaths between arteriosclerotic heart disease and atmospheric cadmium pollution. Occupational exposure to cadmium compounds over extended periods, even in very small quantities, produces kidney damage, an emphysema-like lung disorder, and an apparent lowering of the hemoglobin level of the blood.

Aside from air- and water-borne cadmium compounds that result from mining and industrial operations, the element directly enters the human food chain from cadmium-containing fertilizers and pesticides. Perhaps the highest concentrations have been found in instant coffee (2.27 parts per million), Japanese green tea leaves (2.50 parts per million), beef kidney (12 parts per million), and in lesser quantities in a large variety of sea foods, dairy products, fruits, vegetables, grain products, and oils and fats. In Japan, "Minamata disease" is matched almost by "Itai-Itai" ("It hurts! It hurts!") disease because the patients scream from the pain of cadmium-induced bone disintegration in their bodies. Cadmium salts in large doses, when injected into animals, cause cancer, an association that may also exist between these compounds and humans. Trace quantities of the element may pass through the placental defenses of a pregnant woman and bind to the liver of the fetus. After birth, a breast-fed child acquires an average daily intake of approximately 3.67 micrograms of cadmium per kilogram of body weight from its mother's milk—this, I would add, with a diet of chlorinated hydrocarbons that have been found to exceed the maximum permissible amounts fixed by the FDA for cow's milk.

Even more than lead, mercury, and cadmium, asbestos has had until fairly recently the reputation of being an exclusively occupational hazard. Its harmful effects on workers were noted nearly seventy years ago, when an autopsy on a man who had spent ten years in the carding room of an asbestos textile mill revealed severely scarred lungs that contained numerous asbestos fibers. By the late twenties, this fibrotic syndrome was so well established that it acquired a name of its own, "asbestosis," a disease similar in many ways to silicosis. Asbestos is the general name for a group of hydrated mineral silicates whose fibers can subdivide into fibrils so minute that they can be identified only under an electron microscope. For many years, fire-resistant asbestos minerals were widely used as a construction material and a limited number of industrial products, with the result that their health effects fell largely within the province of industrial medicine. Yet the data that began to accumulate on the potential environmental hazards posed by asbestos were very disquieting. In a widely conducted survey of the early thirties, English researchers reported that as much as 80 percent of asbestos workers who had been employed at their jobs for more than twenty years had symptoms of asbestosis. This shockingly high figure, so suggestive of the mineral's potency in terms of public health, was soon matched by German data, which indicated an equally high percentage of asbestosis among workers who had been exposed for ten years or more. By 1965, one of the most distinguished researchers into asbestos hazards, Irving Selikoff, head of the Environmental Science Laboratory at Mt. Sinai Hospital in New York City, found that of 392 asbestos workers studied in the New York–New Jersey metropolitan area, 339 exhibited unequivocable radiological evidence of asbestosis.

What is even more disturbing, exposure to asbestos is definitely associated in man with a high incidence of cancers of the lung, stomach, colon, rectum, esophagus, and with comparatively rare malignancies, notably cancers of the lung and abdominal cavity linings. Some evidence also exists that occupational exposure to asbestos may play a role in the incidence of intestinal and uterine cancers.

As these studies continued over the years, they began to reveal a very sinister and frightening trend. In the early sixties, J. G. Thomson found that asbestos fibrils were lodged not only in the lungs of workers and people in communities near South African asbestos mines, but also in those living in major cities. By the early seventies, autopsy studies by Selikoff and his associates revealed that nearly half of the lungs examined in New York City had sizable "asbestos bodies" and close to 80 percent contained thin, fine asbestos fibrils. In Finland, surveys conducted between 1960–65 showed that pleural calcification (calcium deposition in the lung cavity lining) occurred in many individuals who lived near asbestos mines. Viewed from almost every aspect—asbestos workers, residents near mines and industrial installations, and the public at large—asbestos was implicated as a causative agent not only in lung fibrosis, but also in a large variety of cancers and a number of pulmonary, gastrointestinal, and possibly brain illnesses. Moreover, the mineral is no longer used merely as a solid fire-proofing agent but in spray form to fire-proof skyscrapers and residential buildings (a form that makes it a very significant atmospheric pollutant), as an inexpensive filler, as floor tiles, paper products, electrical insulation, friction products such as brake linings and clutch facings, asphalt paving, welding-rod coatings, and even as filter media in pharmaceutical products. Twenty to forty years may pass before exposure to asbestos results in cancer. There is no way of knowing what quantities of asbestos may yield a lethal malignancy or how variations in individual responses to large or small "asbestos bodies" may result in cancer.

These "asbestos bodies" are now everywhere in the industrial countries of the world—in the air, water, food chain, and in commonly used materials such as motor vehicles, many paper products, and home construction items. The Reserve Mining Company of Silver Bay, Minnesota, has been dumping 67,000 tons daily of asbestos-laden taconite tailings into once-clear, potable Lake Michigan from which many communities derive their drinking water. In Duluth, Minnesota, a Lake Michigan city with 106,000 people, the high asbestos content of the community's drinking water has caused what amounts to a municipal emergency. By the summer of 1973, the city's residents were warned not to use their water for drinking or cooking. In at least one community center, fountains were shut off to the children. Today, more than a half year after the asbestos problem became a major issue at Duluth, litigation by the federal Environmental Protection Agency has not prevented the mining company from dumping its tailings into the lake or emitting large quantities of asbestos fibers from its smokestacks.

In smaller quantities, the atmosphere has become the dumping ground for industrial metals such as nickel and beryllium, both of which are definitely hazardous, and for low-toxicity metals such as tin, titanium, aluminum, barium, strontium, zirconium, niobium, and vanadium. Although nickel is not nearly as widely distributed in the environment as lead, cadmium, mercury, and asbestos, it causes cancer in humans and animals when inhaled in its carbonyl form. Lung, nose, or sinus cancers among nickel refinery workers are 2 to 25 times higher than we would expect to find in the general population. Continual exposure to beryllium, a highly toxic metal, may cause beryllosis. This disease in its chronic form closely resembles silicosis and leads to progressive loss of respiratory function and eventually to death. Beryllium has long been known as a carcinogenic agent in rats and possibly in humans. The 500-fold increase in the use of beryllium by American industry as an alloy-hardening agent between the late forties and early seventies is making this metal a fairly serious air pollutant.

The emergence of industrial metals, minerals, and compounds as general environmental hazards concretely underscores a broad tendency in modern capitalist society. The entire planet is being reduced to a factory and nature to mere "resources" for reaping extravagant profits. This tendency promotes industrial growth on a scale far beyond the authentic material needs of society, and it systematically fosters irrational "needs" to consume equally irrational products. From the period of the Industrial Revolution onward, we have seen in the factory —with its flat floor, its departmentalization of space, its minute specialization of human labor and thought, and its quantitative criteria of success—the model for our cities and farms. No society prior to the competitive, quantitative, and atomized one in which we live today has so thoroughly devalued contoured space, community, diversity, roundedness of human activity, and qualitative criteria of excellence. That the once strictly occupational diseases of modern industry threaten to become broad public health problems is due not so much to the "proletarianization" of the population as to the total industrialization of nature.

It is a bit too superficial to blame this tendency on the misbehavior, greed, and moral delinquency of a few large corporations, culpable as they may be. On this score, the so-called "radical" wing of the environmentalist "movement" displays more rhetoric than insight. To the degree that Barry Commoner in *The Closing Circle* makes corporate misbehavior a moral problem rather than a tendency inherent in the social system itself, he may have advanced beyond his earlier rather limited technological critique of society, but he still remains far removed from the core problems of the environmental crisis. This crisis is not "somber evidence of an insidious fraud hidden in the vaunted productivity and wealth of modern, technology-based society," as Commoner would have us believe; rather, the crisis is evidence of a marketplace nexus that equates economic survival with growth—a nexus that is perhaps best summarized by the maxim "grow or die."[8] The environmental crisis is inherent in bourgeois society, not in a "modern, technology-based society." It is "somber evidence" not of an "insidious fraud" but of the very law of life of capitalism. It stems not merely from greed but from a market-oriented system in which everything is reduced to a commodity, in which everyone is reduced to a mere buyer or seller, and in which every economic dynamic centers on capital accumulation. Hence the prevailing society is *inherently* antiecological, not only morally delinquent. References to "frauds," "vaunted productivity," and a "modern, technology-based society," however well-intentioned the author's purpose may be, essentially serve to deflect public attention from the deeply social nature of the environmental crisis. A Nadarism that does not reach much beyond judicial litigation and the demand for institutional reforms replaces the historic need for basic social changes.

I do not mean to argue that the objective social factors that daily re-create and extend the environmental crisis leave the corporations morally blameless. Nor do I contend that strong social action must be deferred until we can achieve basic social changes. Rather, I have advanced the view that it is illusory to foster the belief that the environmental crisis is the result of bad intentions; that it can be resolved within the framework of a market economy. Yet we cannot fatalistically bend our knee to the historic eventuality of basic social change while the environment deteriorates before our eyes. The environmental crisis must be attenuated now, as much as possible, if the exploitative practices and zealous "chemo-mania" of an utterly immoral business community, acting in collusion with equally immoral governmental institutions, are not to damage the environment irreparably and expose the public to increasingly hazardous pollutants.

What is most rankling about the behavior of corporate and political interests in the environmental crisis is its all-pervasive hypocrisy. Attacks on "environmental extremists" provide the thinnest veneer for a cynical manipulation of public opinion in behalf of agribusiness, the energy industry, chemical concerns, and major industrial polluters. Where crude propoganda fails, it is followed by outright threats on the part of industry to shut down or relocate installations if "stringent" air and water pollution regulations are not relaxed. Sub rosa attempts are made to sidestep hard-won protective laws for workers and consumers, and massive contributions are made to political campaigns in exchange for privileges and concessions on environmental issues. The extent to which these efforts have become a national scandal makes it unnecessary to belabor them.

What is probably less known, however, is the extent to which environmental and consumer legislation designed to protect the public interest is actually used against it by large corporations, often acting brazenly in collusion with governmental agencies. Means for protecting the consumer become devices for "protecting" industry against the consumer. The "sweeping legislative revisions of [food and drug legislation in] 1958," as I have described them on pages 233–34 of this book, were intended to "make the manufacturer responsible for the safety of a food additive and inserted the Delaney anticancer clause. . . ." In stressing that the 1958 revisions did not flatly prohibit "the use of any toxic chemical additives in food other than those that were clearly indispensable to food production," I did not fully realize how effectively this shortcoming would be used by the FDA and industry against the public interest. Not toxicity as such (the criterion of the earlier law) but "safety," basically a quantitative judgment viewed in terms of "maximum permissible levels," was to guide the admissibility of additives to food.

Although these "sweeping legislative revisions," generally embodied in the Food Additives Amendment of 1958, placed the burden of testing for the safety of a food additive on the manufacturer, they contained an escape clause that recklessly opened a Pandora's box of problems. The amendment cunningly excluded from legislative coverage any substance that is "generally recognized, among experts qualified by scientific training and experience to evaluate its safety, as having been adequately shown through scientific procedures (or, in the case of a substance used in food prior to January 1, 1958, through either scientific procedures or experience based on common use in food) to be safe under the condition of its intended use. . . ."[9]

Accordingly, additives were exempted from the new Food Additives Amendment that, prior to 1958, could be shown on the basis of "experience" to be "safe." Moreover, the FDA acquired the freedom to determine what chemicals were "generally recognized as safe" ("GRAS" chemicals). Here, too, the ambiguity of the words "generally recognized" and "safe" opened the way to highly questionable, if not overtly toxic, food additives that were to provide more than enough fuel for a series of national scandals. In essence, food additives could be used now on the basis of administrative fiat by the FDA and admitted to an elastic "GRAS" list that relied on custom or ("prior to January 1, 1958") on "experience" rather than on sophisticated tests and later experimental study.

Writing at the end of the fifties, shortly after the Food Additives Amendment of 1958 had been passed, I could not have anticipated in *Our Synthetic Environment* how immense this "GRAS" list would become (indeed, one hardly knew it existed when I was writing the book), the administrative scandals it would produce, and the hazards to which it would expose the general public. I had written in *Our Synthetic Environment* that "more than 3,000 chemicals are used in the production and distribution of commercially prepared food." In 1959, when the FDA began to compile a "GRAS" list, the agency listed 189 chemicals. Two years later, in 1961, George P. Larrick, the agency's head, testified before a congressional committee that the list numbered 718 chemicals. By 1964, the figure was officially reported as 575, only to leap to 680 in 1969, according to a report in the Philadelphia *Evening Bulletin*. The term "tested" should be used as elastically as the number of items on the "GRAS" list. According to the most recent data I now have in hand (January 1974), Senator Gaylord Nelson has introduced legislation (S. 2845) that would require that tests be performed on 3,000 approved food additives, none of which has been examined to determine whether it may cause birth defects or genetic damage. This may not be the number of chemicals on the "GRAS" list, but if Nelson's figures are accurate, we have more than traveled full circle since the early sixties if such a stupendous quantity of currently used and FDA-approved food additives has never been tested for such basic features as their mutagenic properties.

Although the very notion of a "GRAS" list had been the target of subterranean criticism for years, the list's contents became the subject of stormy public controversy during the spring and summer of 1969. At that time, John W. Olney of Washington University in St. Louis reported that monosodium glutamate (MSG), a food additive commonly used not only in processed adult foods but also in baby foods caused brain damage in infant mice. Until then, MSG had been honored as a trusted and tried veteran of the "GRAS" list. Industry, which tenderly describes MSG as a "seasoning agent," often adduces it as a "natural product" because it is a compound of glutamic acid, an amino acid normally synthesized by the human body. The FDA had regarded this additive as above reproach. The agency, not to be daunted by any suspicious research results, defended its use with the militancy of a hovering parent whose dearest child has been falsely maligned.

Actually, MSG and glutamic acid are handled quite differently in the bodies of experimental animals. Fed to young rats at 6 percent of diet, MSG reduces growth by as much as 16 percent; by contrast, glutamic acid in similar quantities produces no such effect. A study of MSG, dating as far back as 1957, showed that the "seasoning agent" damages the retinas of newborn animals. Olney, whose findings were published in the spring of 1969, pointed out that the enzymes that help to metabolize MSG in the adult liver do not function as yet in infants and very young animals. With the addition of MSG to the diet, glutamic acid, which normally accumulates in the brain, could easily reach excessive levels in the newly born. In any case, MSG's effect on very young animals, even if injected only during the first few days after birth, are quite dramatic: nerve cells in the hypothalamus swell and die, skeletal growth is stunted, adiposity becomes grotesquely exaggerated, and females become sterile. Such results are found after mice have grown to adulthood, not only in young animals.

No sooner were these grim results given widespread publicity when the integrity of another "GRAS" veteran was demolished. On October 18, 1969, HEW Secretary Robert Finch announced that he was ordering the removal of the artificial sweetener cyclamate from "the list of substances generally recognized as safe for use in foods."[10] That cyclamates could have been placed on the "GRAS" list in the first place in view of mounting evidence that these additives had harmful physiological effects; that they could have been regarded as a "safe" ingredient in generally available foods for individuals of all ages and physical conditions (indeed, some 75 percent of American families were to ingest the "artificial sweetener" before the Finch announcement); that they could have been included in foods and food supplements such as cured bacon and ham, even in children's vitamin pills, without being listed on food labels—all of this is a shuddering commentary on the gross irresponsibility of the food industry, on the pharmaceutical concerns that manufactured cyclamates, and most emphatically, on the higher echelons of the FDA.

Ostensibly, cyclamates were developed originally for people such as diabetics who were placed on a restricted sugar intake. The sweetening agents were marketed in a pill or liquid form under the trade name of Sucaryl and were usually bought in drug stores. Chemically, they were designated as sodium or calcium cyclohexylsulfamate.

They were meant to replace saccharin, which has only a fraction of their "sweetening power," and they produce less of saccharin's metallic taste. According to a standard pharmacology text of the mid-fifties, this "newer sweetening agent" is "practically completely excreted [by the body], and has no known toxicity even after long use, although the total daily dose recommended is only 1.5 Gm."[11]

The most that can be said for this evaluation is that it was unintentionally misleading, although the author might have expressed greater perplexity about so low a "total daily dose" recommendation in a drug that is "practically completely excreted, and has no known toxicity even after long use."[12] Many such evaluations consist largely of descriptions furnished by the manufacturer or by a governmental agency rather than independent research by the author. In fact, the manufacturer, Abbott Laboratories, had filed such an unsatisfactory new drug application for Sucaryl that A. J. Lehman of the FDA described it as "an illustration of how an experiment should not be conducted."[13] Test animals had been too few in number, control groups had been discontinued prematurely, an insufficient number of autopsies had been performed, and the report was too vague to be acceptable. "Abbott's request to market cyclamates would have been rejected," observes James S. Turner in an excellent Nader Study Group report on the FDA, "but the FDA took the unusual position of approving the request on the basis of two-year feeding studies that it had conducted in its own laboratories."[14] Lehman frankly acknowledged that had the FDA not studied cyclamates on its own, he would have been "quite reluctant to permit its use even for drug use, not to mention as an artificial sweetener for foods." As it turned out, the FDA tests revealed "a highly suspicious frequency of lung tumors" and a six-hundred-fold increase in the normal incidence of rare ovarian, kidney, skin, and uterine tumors.[15]

Nevertheless cyclamates were approved for use in diabetic-type foods. This occurred in 1950, eight years before the enactment of the Delaney anticancer clause and a decade or so before the immense promotion campaign launched by the food industry on behalf of dietary beverages and foods for the general public. Despite the most probing congressional investigation of food additives in a generation (the Delaney Committee hearings of the early fifties) and repeated warnings about cyclamates from the Food Nutrition Board of the National Academy of Sciences–National Research Council, the food industry continued to expand the use of cyclamates. In this endeavor, it had the full cooperation of top FDA officials. Ironically, the "GRAS" list and the presence of cyclamates on it completely opened the door to the use of the "sweetening agent" on a lavish scale. The very presence of the agent on the list, a totally arbitrary act by the FDA, was cited by the food industry as evidence of its safety. The "sweetening agent," moreover, could now be used as a cheap substitute for natural sweeteners without disclosing its presence in many staples. Whether consumers wanted to or not, they were unknowingly ingesting cyclamates in many foods and food supplements.

The food industry continued to add cyclamates to foods and beverages on an ever-increasing scale even after 1966 when Japanese researchers reported that the "sweetening agent" could create a clearly hazardous compound, cyclohexylamine, in many bodies. Evidence at hand shows that this transformation occurs in one out of three consumers of cyclamates. Two years later, in March 1968, Jacqueline Verret, an FDA biochemist, came up with a more horrendous piece of evidence. She reported that cyclamates injected into chicken eggs may produce deformities very similar to the grotesque malformations caused by thalidomide. Although this order of evidence was now available to the FDA commissioner and known quite generally to food industry researchers, the advertisements to promote the unrestricted use of cyclamates continued unabated. Absolutely no action was taken on Verret's discovery. In November of the same year, Marvin Legator, the FDA's cell biology research chief, found that cyclohexylamine, the compound formed from cyclamates in the bodies of many consumers, is a mutagenic agent. It breaks, in Legator's words, "a significant number of chromosomes in both *in vitro* and *in vivo* animal studies."[16] The efforts by FDA chieftains to sidestep these appalling facts discovered by the agency's own researchers provide incredible reading in Turner's account. Here, it suffices merely to note that Legator's memorandum on his research, emphatically concluding that the use of cyclamates "should be immediately curtailed, pending the outcome of additional studies," was deleted by a cabal of his superiors. "Without informing Dr. Legator, Dr. Banes [to whom Dr. Legator's memo was addressed], or Commissioner Ley," notes Turner, "a new memorandum was prepared and forwarded over Dr. Legator's name with the same heading and date, using the original language, but omitting the strong recommendation against cyclamate use."[17] Turner describes this behavior as a "deceptive" action.

Cyclamates were not banned for use in food until evidence emerged in 1969 that the "sweetening agents" cause bladder cancer in rats. It was on these grounds alone that Finch, with obvious reluctance and with cynical asides against the Delaney anticancer clause, removed the agents from the "GRAS" list. Later, by deferring the execution of the ban from February 1,

1970 (as originally announced) to September 1 and by excluding beverages from the ban, HEW gave industry every opportunity to clear its shelves and warehouses of this extremely hazardous compound. These deferrals, restrictions, and retreats from the original, more sweeping ban of October 1969, were made in total disregard of mounting evidence that cyclamates were not only carcinogenic but also mutagenic agents. Furthermore, there is reason to suspect that cyclamates disrupt the effect of anticoagulants in humans, perhaps adversely affect the way in which certain drugs bind to blood plasma, cause softening of the stool, cross the placentas of pregnant women, reach infants through their mothers' milk, and so forth, ad nauseum.

Turner's conclusions about the way in which Finch, presumably one of Nixon's more "liberal" cabinet officers, dealt with the cyclamate problem and the issues his behavior raised are worth citing in full:

When HEW Secretary Robert H. Finch finally removed cyclamates from the GRAS list and the market, he too did not mention the doubts contained in fifteen years of scientific writing about the chemical. He misled and confused the American public. He did not warn that scientific knowledge about chemical hazards is severely limited. He did not try to explain that the law requires a food additive to be established as safe before it is used and that the manufacturer of cyclamates had failed to meet this responsibility. Instead he chose to dismiss all but one narrow study suggesting a connection between rat cancer and cyclamates. Rather than clearly asserting his authority, the Secretary backed into an apologetic enforcement of one particular codicil of the law, saying, "I have acted under the provisions of the law because . . . I am required to do so." The Secretary's press conference and his subsequent actions suggest that he misunderstands the 1958 Food Additive Amendment and the hazards it was meant to control. He seemed to consider it unimportant that an additive be proven safe before it was cleared for use in food, and he appeared willing to permit modification of the law to allow distribution in food of elements that had not been proven safe. He spoke of the growing scientific concern about the increasing number of chemicals that individuals come in contact with as if it were insignificant. He treated as unnecessary the protection of every scientist's right to communicate his findings to his fellow scientists and the general public.[18]

Clearly, Turner's remarks do not apply to Finch alone. They characterize decades of food and drug administration in which the public interest was shamelessly ignored in behalf of vested corporate interests. As Turner correctly observes, what is basically at issue in the food additives problem (and the pollution problem generally, I might add) can be posed in a simple pragmatic question: "when a food additive presents a possible risk, shall it be allowed in the food supply until proven unsafe, or shall it be excluded from the food supply until proven safe? In other words, shall the safety of a food additive be tested in human beings or in rats? In the case of cyclamates, the position of the FDA has amounted to a belief that the testing should be done on people. If the food industry can use a questionable additive until it is conclusively proven to be unsafe, people will be injured."[19]

The many additives and pollutants I've adduced thus far do not exhaust the evidence that supports Turner's damning conclusions. That agribusiness, industry, and the FDA have learned almost nothing from the MSG and cyclamate crises of 1969 is clearly revealed by the vacillation they have shown in later situations and by very recent evidence of widely used food additives that are as hazardous as the cyclamates. The FDA's indecision in dealing with brominated vegetable oils, which Canadian experimenters as early as 1968 found to be causal factors in producing heart damage, retarded growth, digestive difficulties, liver and kidney enlargement, and spleen and thyroid damage in rats; the agency's on-again, off-again approach toward FD&C Red No. 4, a highly suspicious coal-tar dye, which was banned on suspicion of producing serious bladder damage in rats and later rehabilitated for use as a dye in maraschino cherries; a similar vacillating approach in dealing with phosphate detergents, which not only promote rampant algal growth, with its consequent pollution of waterways, but also contain appreciable quantities of arsenic—all of these fairly recent episodes are evidence of more than institutional naïvete or scientific myopia. In connection with the FDA's "vacillations" on cyclamates, Turner quotes one perplexed FDA laboratory assistant as noting: "It makes you wonder about the agency. It all seems like politics, not science." Perhaps a more appropriate word would be "economics," or more bluntly—"profit, not science."[20]

The most recent research reveals that other veteran additives may be even more harmful than cyclamates. Nitrates, which have been used for generations to brighten the color (and conceal the fat content) of processed meats, may not only turn into nitrites in the body and bind with hemoglobin to diminish a consumer's oxygen supply, they may also combine with amines in the stomach to form highly carcinogenic nitrosamines. Although these data were known to the food industry and the FDA since the summer of 1973, supermarkets are replete with frankfurters, sausages, packaged bacon, ham, beef products, and the like that contain not only sodium nitrate but also sodium nitrite.

What is no less disquieting, vinyl chloride, a widely used compound for producing plastic polyvinyl chloride, is suspected of causing an appalling increase in the incidence of a rare, invariably fatal liver cancer. Normally, this form of cancer claims only twenty-five lives a year; as of February 1974, six Goodrich workers who were exposed to vinyl chloride in the firm's Louisville, Kentucky, plant died of the disease. Authorized for use as food and beverage containers by the FDA in 1969, polyvinyl chloride plastics have long been an object of suspicion. In the summer of 1973, the agency placed a temporary ban on the use of these containers for liquor. The containers had been employed over various periods, in some cases for as long as four years, by some thirty American distillers. Residues as high as 20 parts per million of vinyl chloride had been found in liquor stored in the plastic bottles. Close to a billion polyvinyl chloride containers have been produced in the United States. It remains to determine how extensively such containers are used for foods and beverages generally and to what extent public health is endangered by the polyvinyl chloride in paints, construction pipes, furniture, upholstery, draperies, wall coverings, floor tiles, tablecloths, toys, clothing, footwear, garden hoses, phonograph records, dentures, and pharmaceutical products.

I have not listed this detailed variety of products, to which hundreds of millions of people are exposed, to be facetious. On the average, every American ingests three to four pounds of food additives a year. These are the more than 3,000 "intentional additives" which the food industry uses at an annual expenditure variously estimated from $300 to $500 million to color, soften, plasticize, flavor, preserve, homogenize, and otherwise "modify" the quality and appearance of food. A substantial portion of these food additives misleads the consumer into thinking she or he is acquiring a "fresher," more "nutritious," and generally "healthier" product. In fact, many of these additives simply replace natural nutrients by cheap, often nutritively inferior and nonnutritive (when not outrightly toxic) ingredients whose unconscionable function is to increase the profits of the manufacturer. To the 3,000 "intentional additives," we must add an incalculable number of "unintentional additives," substantial quantities of which are discovered every year, such as vinyl chlorides in liquor. How much of a burden many of these carcinogenic, mutagenic, and generally hazardous additives place on the human body is veiled in obscurity.

Some indication of what this overall burden may produce in human beings was suggested by expert testimony last spring at hearings of the Senate Select Committee on Nutrition and Human Needs. According to Ben Feingold, chairman emeritus of the Kaiser-Permanente Medical Center allergy division, there is convincing evidence that the artificial colors and flavors used in nearly all of our processed foods cause hyperactivity in children. "We can turn these kids on and off at will simply by regulating their diets," observed Feingold. "There is no reason not to wonder whether food additives affect adult emotional behavior as well."[21]

The perversion of the American diet by its profit-hungry "servant," the food and beverage industry, is no longer an indictment leveled by what the FDA normally labels "quacks" and "crackpots." In the ruthless prose of Daniel Zwerdling: "Scary stories about the risks of eating are now coming from well-known and sober university deans and government scientists. Ten of them appeared quietly before the Senate Select Committee on Nutrition and Human Needs last spring to testify that our daily diets of processed foods, rich in refined sugar and modified carbohydrates like white flour, are probably major causes of diabetes, heart and arterial disease, and intestinal cancer—among other ailments. Most eaters don't like to believe this or to connect their lunch to a disease that will kill them fifteen years from now. So the hearings didn't make the headlines as the political scandals did. . . ."[22] Perhaps Mr. Zwerdling's conclusion would have been closer to the truth if he gave greater recognition to high advertising expenditures of the $161 billion per year food and beverage industry in American newspapers, radio, and television.

According to Senator Charles Percy in his opening statement before the committee, Americans consume 21 to 25 percent fewer dairy products, vegetables, and fruits than they did two decades ago and 70 to 80 percent more junk food, such as soft drinks and sugary snacks. "Most Americans now eat more processed and synthetic food," observes Zwerdling, "than the real thing." This dietary regimen, worse by far than I could have anticipated a dozen years ago, has left us with an adult population nearly half of which is overweight or grossly fat. It has produced a significant portion that, according to one federal survey (aborted by the Nixon administration when its preliminary results seemed too embarrassing), "was malnourished or was at high risk of developing nutritional problems."[23] Typically, the average American adult now consumes 126 pounds of sugar a year and children consume considerably more. This single statistic, an increase of more than 25 percent over the conservative data I adduced twelve years ago, quantitatively measures the deterioration of the American diet from the low level that already appalled so many of my readers when *Our Synthetic Environment* was first published.

Environmentally, we are a beleaguered species—not by natural forces that inflict material scarcity and toil as unavoidable features of the human condition, but by social forces that create irrational relations and requirements as utterly needless features of our lifeways. From the maze of statistics and data that fully reveal these irrationalities, space limitations make it possible to select only a few, almost at random, that bear witness to the whole. Our air is now so polluted that carbon monoxide, which as I noted earlier was almost dismissed a decade ago as a trifling problem, is now singled out as one of the most serious threats to public health. *Item*: A nationwide survey of nearly 30,000 blood donors by Wisconsin researchers in eighteen areas of the United States between 1969–72 revealed (in the words of the report) "the astounding observation that 45 percent of all nonsmoking blood donors tested had carbon monoxide saturations greater than 1.5 percent," that is, greater than the highest safe level for active nonsmokers established by the 1971 Clean Air Act's quality standards. "None of the large urban centers had carbon monoxide concentrations low enough to comply with the Environmental Protection Agency ambient air quality standards for carbon monoxide."[24] The data so appalled the researchers that they seriously questioned the wisdom of transfusing blood donated by a smoker, who might be expected to have even higher carbon monoxide blood concentrations than a nonsmoker, to patients with serious cardiovascular disease.

Our waterways are now so polluted that we are faced with a return of traditional bacterial and viral epidemics that public health movements of the last century had resolved generations ago. *Item*: A national survey of impure tap water by Gladwin Hill, one of *The New York Times*'s most prestigious reporters, in May 1973, cited EPA warnings "that despite the widespread assumption in space-age America that impeccable drinking water can be taken for granted, such deplorable conditions exist among the nation's water systems that there are countless places where a grave epidemic might occur any day." Mr. Hill referred not only to mercury, lead, and asbestos poisoning or to "the 12,000 toxic chemicals now used in industry with hundreds of new compounds being added each year . . . many of which find their way into water sources"; nor was he concerned only with the insecticides, herbicides, and nitrites that are saturating American waterways.[25] He was concerned also with salmonellosis, hepatitis, and typhoid epidemics—and had he chosen not to be "alarmist," he might have added cholera epidemics of which serious outbreaks recently occurred in western Europe. Indeed, a survey of nearly 1,000 public water systems revealed that over 40 percent deliver water of inferior quality and 36 percent contain bacteria or chemicals exceeding safe limits. According to Jay H. Lehr, executive director of the National Water Well Association, recent surveys clearly show "our drinking water supplies to be in horrible shape."[26]

The development of huge metropolitan centers in the United States, of immense urban belts that form the environment for nearly 70 percent of the American people, has produced problems of waste disposal that form a major crisis within the environmental crisis as a whole. *Item*: A recent study by the National League of Cities and the United States Conference of Mayors, released in mid-1973, reveals that cities are beset with the disposing of 250 million tons of trash a year. This trash consists of 28 billion bottles, 48 billion cans, 4 million tons of plastic, 30 million tons of paper, 100 million tires, and over 30 million junk cars. New York City alone generates 30,000 tons of solid wastes a day, most of which is either burned, used as land fill, or dumped into nearby Atlantic waters where it mixes with sewage and industrial wastes from the metropolitan area. Quite recently, scientists studying the waters off Long Island's south shore, a resort area regarded as one of the finest in the world, discovered a lifeless marine area formed by a long accumulation of sludge, which the city has discharged at the rate of 5 million cubic yards a year—enough to cover an area as large as Central Park. This dead sea occupies twenty-five square miles and, contrary to the initial anticipations that followed its discovery, it is very much on the move. From a distance of ten miles off Long Island, it has moved to within a half mile of the island's beaches. Divers describe these lifeless waters as "black as pitch," indeed so inky that the blackness is impenetrable to a powerful underwater flashlight.

These immense metropolitan areas are sources not only of massive air, water, and solid-waste pollution but also of harmful stress conditions and damaging noise levels. Noise levels in the range of 80 decibels distinctly contribute to hearing impairment. At 70 decibels or more, noise can accelerate the heart beat, change breathing patterns, increase the motility of the gastrointestinal tract, and alter secretions of saliva and gastric juices. According to Samuel Rosen, a specialist in the physiological effects of noise, the high noise levels commonly encountered in urban environments raise blood cholesterol concentrations in laboratory animals, cause heart enlargement, increase adrenal hormone secretion, heighten blood pressure, and significantly constrict blood vessels. The suspicion is growing that continual exposure to noise levels in major urban areas contributes materially to the incidence and exacerbation of cardiovascular and mental disorders. *Item*: A survey last year of Montreal noise levels (a relatively quiet city by comparison with American cities of similar size and population) revealed that the downtown area produces background noise levels of 80 decibels, reaching nearly 90 decibels during relatively light midmorning highway traffic, and soaring to over 100 decibels at construction sites where jack hammers are used. Environmental Protection Agency surveys indicate that exposure to noise from a heavy truck or a pneumatic drill for eight hours at a distance of 50 feet will damage hearing. The noise produced by a New York City subway takes us into the 100 decibel range, where it is distinctly harmful to riders at all levels—from their hearing to their physiological and psychological well-being.

If we look beyond the specific pollutants and pollution episodes that feed the muckracking environmental literature of our time to the broader issues of ecological balance, our present practices can only be interpreted as an unprecedented socionatural crisis of staggering dimensions. During the thirties, it could have been argued with some plausibility that our environmental problems were more pharmacological than ecological; that we were endangered by acutely toxic poisons, not by profound imbalances between humanity and nature—hidden as these imbalances surely were at the time. But they were not evident, and the term "ecology" was still an esoteric word. This was the era of Kallet and Schlink's *100 Million Guinea Pigs*, an immensely popular book that read more like a text on toxicology than ecology. Mass production of food had yet to reach the dimensions it has today—together with the supermarket and shopping center. Food production was still to a great extent a local, rather decentralized activity; hence, a dangerous pollutant or additive affected a smaller consuming population than it does today. Cities, while wretchedly polluted in many areas, were more definable and smaller. Los Angeles, for example, had yet to experience serious smog problems. New York's air was relatively clear, and while industrial areas were shrouded in "smoke," the exotic poisons that multiply yearly in the environment—often tasteless and unrecognizable to their victims—were com-

paratively few in number and reached smaller populations than they do at present.

What now confronts us are not only the specific, often
easily degradable toxicants of two generations ago, but
the long-lived carcinogens and mutagens such as chlorinated hydrocarbons, industrial metals, hazardous components of plastics, and radioactive isotopes. These
dangerous agents do not necessarily produce acute symptoms, nor are they quickly degraded into harmless components by the body or the natural environment. To the
contrary, they last for very long periods of time and become part of the individual's very anatomy, entering her
or his bone structure and fat depots, where they silently
accumulate without any overt effects for years. Slowly
they undermine the general health, well-being, and
longevity of people in immense numbers, often culmi-
nating in disabling chronic diseases, psychic disorders,
congenital malformations, and cancers. Their toxic effects
may not be seen until decades have passed. They produce
harm to the body not only in large quantities but also in
trace amounts. Our senses do not easily perceive them,
nor are many of them detectable even by conventional
analytic techniques. They imperceptibly damage not only
specific individuals and segments of the population but
also the entire human species, indeed, the entire world
of life.

Today we must reconsider seriously what we mean
by a "pollutant." In the 1930s it would have seemed
ridiculous to call heat or carbon dioxide a "pollutant,"
and terms like "thermal pollution" would have been as
incomprehensible as the word "ecology." Yet now carbon
dioxide and heat may rank among the most serious
sources of ecological disequilibrium. Modern industrial
and domestic combustion activities emit carbon dioxide
in such enormous amounts that the gas has increased

in the atmosphere by roughly 25 percent over the past 100 years and may well double again by the year 2000. Contemporary readers need not be reminded in detail about the "greenhouse effect"; the gas, it is supposed, by inhibiting the dissipation of the earth's heat into space, will eventually cause the polar ice caps to melt and thereby lead to the inundation of vast coastal and low-lying areas. As for thermal pollution, the result primarily of warm water discharged by conventional and nuclear power plants, its effects on the ecology of lakes, rivers, and estuaries have received so much publicity that it hardly requires discussion. It suffices merely to point out that lakes and waterways have become stagnant sewers owing to the algal blooms produced by the heat, not to speak of the damage inflicted on fish life.

Pollution has now become so widespread, so complex, and so lasting owing to the durability of the new pollutants that it threatens to undermine the biogeochemical cycles on which we depend for an ecologically viable planet. Agribusiness not only diminishes the nutritive capacity of soil with its exploitative industrial techniques, but its profligate use of highly soluble, inorganic nitrogen fertilizers affects the nitrogen cycle itself, just as our mindless combustion of fossil fuels affects the carbon and oxygen cycles. Hydrological cycles are being undermined by the exploitation and pollution of water resources. Owing to our overuse of ground water and other underground fluids, cities like Tokyo and Los Angeles are subsiding by several inches each year. The draining of water reserves from ecologically precarious arid regions produces an ever-greater infusion of salt water and threatens to ruin fertile agricultural areas irreparably. Estuaries and coastal shallows, which form the spawning grounds for some of our most valuable aquatic food animals, are being destroyed by water pollutants and land fills; salt marshes, which provide rich feeding and breeding grounds for wildfowl, are being drained or otherwise eliminated for real estate developments. Our congested cities are altering the climate of the regions they occupy as well as eating into invaluable fertile land.

Defoliation has now ruined immense areas of Vietnam for a century or more. Some of the herbicides employed in the war are currently used in agriculture abroad and are almost certainly known to be mutagenic agents. After years of use, they have been diffused widely all over the planet. Surface mining has horribly disfigured immense areas of the world (not only the United States) and threatens to eat away ever-larger areas as the myth of the "energy crisis" is manipulated to undermine the limited environmental restrictions that have been placed on the energy industry. Underground nuclear tests have reactivated ancient geological faults and exposed populated areas to the danger of catastrophic earthquakes. "Breaks in rocks caused by such explosions normally are not visible from the surface," observes Thomas Detwyler of the University of Michigan, "although a test in Nevada in 1968 (ironically named the Faultless test) created a long surface fault with a virtual displacement of 15 feet."[27] J. H. Healy and his colleagues of the National Center for Earthquake Research warn that the injection of fluids into basement rock, whether to store lethal wastes or to compensate for withdrawals of underground liquids, triggers seismic activity.

Truly global in its effect is the pollution of the oceans —a phenomenon so widespread that even remote Arctic waters are reported to resemble cesspools and have suffered a measurable decline in plankton population, the tiny plants and animals that comprise the starting point for all aquatic food chains. Since the wreck of the *Torrey Canyon* off the coast of Cornwall in 1967 and the

Santa Barbara drilling leakage of 1969, we have become
acutely aware of the enormous damage marine life has
suffered from oil pollution. With tanker sizes burgeoning
from less than 20,000 deadweight tons in 1930 to 800,000
in the 1970s, future spillages are likely to be even more
catastrophic. These episodes, however, tend to obscure
the daily "spillages," often deliberate washouts, of tankers
and other vessels that introduce millions of gallons of oil
into the marine environment. Sizable oil slicks have been
found at every latitude. The short-term effects of these
oil spills have been dramatically illustrated by photo-
graphs of dead and dying sea birds, but the long-term
effects, as Max Blumer of the Woods Hole Oceanographic
Institution warns, may be less obvious but more sinister.
Ironically, it is "likely that the treatment of oil spills
with detergents or dispersants, or the natural dispersion
of oil in storms, produces oil droplets of a particle size
range that is ingested and assimilated by many marine
organisms. Once assimilated, this oil passes through the
marine food chain and eventually reaches organisms that
are harvested for human consumption."[28] Perhaps the
most serious effect of this process, Blumer warns, "is the
potential accumulation in human food of long-term poisons derived from crude oil, for instance, of carcinogenic
compounds."[29]

   In all of these cases, we are distorting and under-
mining the most fundamental cycles necessary for the
integrity of the biosphere. There is no historic precedent
to equal the impact of the prevailing irrational society on
nature, even in a period as brief as the one which followed
World War II. By comparison, the prewar era seems almost pristine in its behavior, however savagely it raped
the North American continent and other areas of the
world. True, the natural world's recuperative powers
should not be discounted; the biosphere has survived

tremendous catastrophes in the past—ice ages, epochal climatic changes, major shifts in wind and rainfall patterns that have totally dessicated once-luxuriant areas, and seismic activity that profoundly changed the face of entire continents. These severe shocks imposed by nature itself, far from destroying the world of life, served in many ways to foster its development toward a greater diversity of forms, flexibility of adaptive and survival mechanisms, and the elaboration of increasingly intelligent behavior patterns. The resiliency of the biosphere in dealing with damage caused by modern society is cause for considerable hope; it may well provide us with the lead time to rework our social relationships along lines that will serve to harmonize our relationships with nature. A paralyzing "doomsday syndrome," to use John Maddox's phrase, that leads to hopeless fatalism in the face of an unalterable social tendency toward immolation could be as harmful as a roseate optimism that naïvely preens itself on a mindless commitment to "progress" and "growth."[30]

Nor can we place this "doomsday syndrome" in the service of a social dilettantism that holds either technology as such or some abstract "we" responsible for the natural imbalances produced by an inherently irrational society. In recent years a type of biological "cold warrior" has emerged who tends to locate the ecological crisis in technology and population growth, thereby divesting it of its explosive social content. Out of this focus has emerged a new version of "original sin" in which tools and machines, reinforced by sexually irresponsible humans, ravage the earth in concert. Both technology and sexual irresponsibility, so the argument goes, must be curbed— if not voluntarily, then by the divine institution called the state.

The naïvete of this approach would be laughable

were it not for its sinister implications. History has known
of many different forms of tools and machines: some of
which are patently harmful to human welfare and the
natural world, others of which have clearly improved the
condition of humanity and the ecology of an area. It
would be absurd to place plows and mutagenic defoliants,
weaving machines and automobiles, computers and moon
rockets, under a common rubric. Worse, it would be
grossly misleading to deal with these technologies in a
social vacuum.

Technologies consist not only of the devices humans
employ to mediate their relationships with the natural
world but also the attitudes associated with these devices.
These attitudes are distinctly social products, the results
of social relationships humans establish with each other.
What is clearly needed is not a mindless deprecation of
technology as such, but rather a reordering and rede-
velopment of technologies according to ecologically sound
principles. We need an ecotechnology, based on nonpol-
luting energy sources, such as solar and wind power,
methane generators, and possibly liquid hydrogen, that
will harmonize society with the natural world.

The same oversimplification is evident in the neo-
Malthusian alarm over population growth. The reduction
of population growth to a mere ratio between birth rates
and death rates obscures the many complex social factors
that enter into both statistics. A rising or declining birth
rate is not a simple biological datum, any more than a
rising or declining death rate. Both are subject to the
influences of the economic status of the individual, the
nature of the family, the values of society, the status of
women, the social attitudes toward children, the culture of
the community, and so forth. A change in any single factor
interacts with the remainder to produce the statistical
data called "birth rates" and "death rates." Culled from

such abstract ratios, population growth rates can easily be used to foster authoritarian controls and finally a totalitarian society, especially if neo-Malthusian propaganda and the failure of voluntary birth control are used as an excuse. In arguing that forcible measures of birth control and a calculated policy of indifference to hunger may eventually be necessary to stabilize world populations, the neo-Malthusians are already creating a climate of opinion that will make genocidal policies and authoritarian institutions socially acceptable.

Today, what should be of greater ecological concern to us than the population growth rates of India are the soaring production rates of the United States. The increased output of useless, shoddy, even hazardous goods designed to meet irrational "needs" is clearly demonstrated by the fact that nearly 10 percent of American industrial capacity is committed to military production. Immense quantities of cheaply made ephemeral material are manufactured that constitute an almost unabashed waste of resources; this staggering output, in turn, leaves behind mountains of rubbish that must be disposed of in some manner. At both ends of the spectrum, from production through consumption to disposal, these commodities place an immense burden on global ecology. By contrast with the industrial and political managers of the prevailing antiecological society, the public has shown an intuitive decency that stands sharply at odds with the neo-Malthusian image of the human species, an image of humanity as so many fruit flies that will multiply indefinitely until (in the language of the population literature) there will be "no standing room." If birth rates today are declining in the United States and in the Western world generally, this is not because Paul Ehrlich's *Population Bomb* and similar works have had a decisive ideological impact. The sources for this demographic reversal can best be found, I believe, in the changing sexual mores introduced by the counterculture of the sixties and the new conceptions women are forming of their roles as human beings. Similarly, mounting public concern over the hazards posed by air and water pollution, synthetic foods, and nuclear power plants has done far more to reduce or at least decelerate the damage inflicted on the environment than all the pious speeches delivered by "eco"-politicians and governmental bureaucrats. To the degree that environmentalists deal with social problems as strictly biological ones—to the extent that they analogize human population fluctuations to the proliferation of *Drosophila* and house flies—and perhaps more sinisterly, to the extent that they create a ubiquitous "we" that equates the behavior of materially insecure workers with their overly affluent employers, ghetto blacks with suburban whites, oppressed women with domineering males—environmentalism tends to become the reactionary handmaiden of the industrial, financial, and political bandits who rule this society. The more recent gospel of "scarcity" generated by a cynically contrived "energy crisis" and by calculated shortages of vital materials serves more to validate windfall profits for oil corporations and the subversion of environmentalist restrictions on an industrial apparatus gone mad than to promote sound ecological practices in dealing with the natural world. The alternatives confronting us today are not between energy shortages and scarcity, but between an irrational system of production and a society based on ecological principles, one that can amply meet rational human needs with a minimum of onerous toil. We can have all the energy we need if we use the sun and wind rather than fossil and nuclear fuels. We can have all the material amenities of life if we produce goods of lasting quality and if we rescale our needs along humanistic lines. To make these sweeping

changes implies an entirely new social order in which the
planet is shared communally by free people with a non-
hierarchical, cooperative mentality, rather than parceled
out privately as so much real estate to satisfy competitive,
profit-oriented egotists.

Although criticizing a "doomsday syndrome" that
leads to passive fatalism, I do not wish to understate the
gravity of the present ecological crisis and the global
disaster the prevailing society will almost certainly produce if it is permitted to run its course. Indeed, on one
score—the growing problem of public exposure to ionizing radiation and the proliferation of nuclear energy
power plants—a "doomsday syndrome," provided it does
not abort militant public action, is more relevant than
the radiant optimism exuded by governmental agencies
and the energy industry. I have no reason to mute the
alarm *Our Synthetic Environment* sounded on the risks
posed by diagnostic X-radiation, although this area has
been marked by considerable improvement. New York,
New Jersey, and California now require that X-ray technicians be properly trained and certified. The heightened
awareness reflected by these regulations, together with
increased periodic inspections of X-ray equipment, augers
well for a more rational and prudent use of radiation for
diagnostic and therapeutic purposes. Yet the problem is
still with us, and Karl Z. Morgan, director of the Health
Physics Division of the Oak Ridge National Laboratory,
has estimated as recently as 1971 that medical uses of
X-radiation may claim as many as 27,000 genetic and
leukemic deaths annually in the United States. This
figure is admittedly on the high side of Morgan's estimates, but it does not include thyroid and bone cancers
induced by diagnostic X-radiation, which may number
as many as 1,000 annually. In other respects, since the
publication of *Our Synthetic Environment*, public ex-

posure to radiation has been increased by defective color television sets and the use of high-voltage vacuum switches in industries, hospitals, and universities that have been known to reach two million times the permissible nonoccupational rate at one foot from the switch. The use of cement blocks for home construction made from Conasauga shale and phosphate rock, minerals that contain high concentrations of uranium ores, may well be exposing families in such homes to radon gas, a daughter product of uranium decay. Radon, a highly dangerous radioactive element that has so appreciably increased the incidence of lung cancer in uranium miners, may produce similar effects in ordinary families who unknowingly live in homes made of uranium-rich material.

X-ray machines and high-voltage vacuum switches, of course, can be turned off. Once this happens, they are harmless. And when these devices are in operation, their use can be carefully regulated. Even uranium-rich building materials can be restored to areas from which they were acquired; unless they are extracted from below the surface, they do not add significantly to natural background levels of radiation to which all life-forms have adapted over millions of years. But the wastes produced by nuclear reactors represent an entirely different problem. Most of them did not exist in any appreciable quantities before the "atomic age"; some are entirely man-made and represent biological unknowns for all living species. Already our planet is burdened by very large, easily diffused concentrations of reactor wastes whose potential for damage is described in some detail in this book. Existing wastes contained in the large storage tanks of the Atomic Energy Commission will be with humanity for centuries to come. Nothing can diminish the lethal activity of these wastes but the passage of time. Society's only protection from the mutagenic, carcinogenic, and physically debilitating effects of alpha, beta, and gamma radiation is its ability to shield effectively the emitters from the public.

Among nuclear technicians, both the critics and supporters of expanded nuclear power programs, the debate over the wisdom of nuclear power plants tends to center around the possibility of serious accidents. There is general agreement that a "burner reactor" (one that operates by the straightforward fissioning of our very limited supplies of uranium-235) does not develop the kind of critical mass that occurs in nuclear weapons. These plants cannot explode like an atomic bomb. Accordingly, the most serious kind of accident that could occur in a burner reactor would be a meltdown: its fuel elements would become overheated and begin to fuse into a molten radioactive mass. Assuming that the reactor's emergency coolant supply failed to arrest this process, the uranium fuel and its fission products would form a glowing ball weighing 100 tons, which could melt through the 6- to 8-inch carbon steel containment vessel in about a half hour, penetrate the surrounding 3- to 4-foot-thick reinforced concrete and steel liner before the end of a day, and finally release an incalculable quantity of deadly fission products into the environment.

To AEC spokesmen, accidents of this kind are not impossible; they are simply "highly improbable." According to these gentlemen, the "odds" against any "serious accident" ranges around the order of "10,000 to 1." This type of argument and the numbers game behind it have a history of its own. Seventeen years ago, the AEC had calculated the hazards of an accident on the basis of the "worst case" that could occur. Critics of the agency's nuclear reactor program could plausibly demonstrate with the AEC's own data that the ever-increasing size of reactors over the years increased the possibility of accidents and the deadly damage they could inflict. With the appointment of James Schlesinger as head of the AEC in the summer of 1971, the agency's views on this subject underwent a marked philosophical change. Schlesinger, now Mr. Nixon's secretary of defense, essentially decided that estimates of accidents were to be based not on the "worst case," but on the "best engineering judgment." In the words of Norman Rasmussen of MIT, who charted this new formulation into an AEC guideline: "Uncertainties are treated by developing realistic probability values of all possible outcomes rather than choosing the worst possible values. . . . This should provide a more complete and accurate view of nuclear accident risks than previous studies that computed only 'worst case' values." Thus the grave hazards involved in building nuclear plants near densely populated communities and the full implications of a meltdown by a runaway reactor were semantically glossed over by a "probablistic approach."[31] This approach made a terrifying disaster, which might kill or gravely injure immense numbers of people, neither "terrifying" nor "disastrous," but statistically "improbable."

What would be the biological results of a runaway meltdown—even if, as the AEC claims, the chances that it could occur are 10,000 to 1? If an accident of this kind occurred near a large metropolitan area, hundreds of thousands of people would be exposed to lethal dosages of radiation. As Henry W. Kendall, a high-energy physicist at MIT who has served as a Nader advisor, observes: "The radioactive accumulation in a large power reactor is equivalent to the fallout from thousands of Hiroshima-size nuclear weapons. . . . Consider, for example, that 20 percent of a reactor's radioactive material is gaseous in normal circumstances and, if released to the environment in one way or another, could be swept along by the winds for many tens of miles to expose people outside the reactor site boundaries to what could be lethal amounts of radioactivity. The lethal distance may approach 100 miles."[32]

However small the odds may be that this kind of accident will occur, the fact remains that it *might* occur. The AEC's nuclear reactor program could never confer enough benefits to allow us to turn this risk into a reality. In any case, much of the agency's discussions around the "probable odds" are essentially unreliable guesswork. They are based not on practical test experiences but on highly dubious computer models. A loss-of-coolant-accident test, based on pipe breakages in a 9-inch-diameter reactor model, revealed to everyone's embarrassment that the emergency coolant designed to prevent a complete meltdown simply flowed through the break in the coolant pipe. The emergency coolant never affected the reactor core.

Neither the doubts of its critics nor the questionable data at its disposal deterred the AEC from proposing the construction of the world's largest nuclear reactor of its day (1962) a few hundred yards away from the United Nations buildings. More recently, the agency tried to promote the building of reactors on marine platforms off Coney Island and the New Jersey coast. It approved the siting of three large nuclear reactors at Indian Point, just twenty-six miles north of New York City. As reactors get larger and larger, they are being constructed closer and closer to the large cities of the United States. The safety of high density areas is being traded away for the profitability that electric utilities gain from close proximity to their markets. Despite the AEC's extravagant assurances that the nuclear reactors are well-constructed and safe, the equipment that arrives on site is often so faulty and so shoddily manufactured that the agency's ambitious plans to expand its energy programs have been aborted by shutdowns, the need to rerate output, and unexpected releases of radioactivity into the environment. The unreliability of nuclear power plants "is becoming one of their most dependable features," observes Thomas Ehrich in a survey of the problem for *The Wall Street Journal.* "The incredibly complex facilities are plagued by breakdowns that experts blame on faulty engineering, defective equipment and operating errors. Failures range from hour-long annoyances to months-long closedowns. Repair costs often run into millions of dollars and some utilities stoically shell out up to $200,000 a day for replacement electricity to distribute to their customers."[33]

Yet in the long run, the greatest hazard of the AEC's nuclear reactor program lies not so much in its potential for serious accidents as in the enormous accumulation of highly radioactive reactor wastes the reactors produce. These wastes do not differ very significantly in kind from the radioactive material produced by nuclear weapons explosions. My account of the radioactivity generated by bomb tests in *Our Synthetic Environment,* its entry into the food chain, and its biological effects is as relevant today as it was twelve years ago. Indeed, the situation described in my chapter on this subject is potentially worse than it was in the early sixties. Some thirty nuclear power plants are currently on-stream in the United States. Plans exist to expand this figure to one thousand by the end of the century. It is almost impossible to consider the immense problems humanity will face for centuries to come in trying to deal with the handling, transportation, storage, and surveillance of this lethal material. Merely from burner reactors alone that fission uranium-235, future generations will inherit a precarious legacy that may produce incalculable damage to the biosphere.

But uranium-235 comprises less than 1 percent of the world's more substantial uranium reserves, notably the relatively plentiful but nonfissionable isotope uranium-238. The future of the burner reactor is thus limited, possibly to little more than a generation or two. The future of the nuclear reactor program lies in developing "breeders"—reactors that convert plentiful uranium-238 into fissionable plutonium-239. Far from diminishing the waste problems which burner reactors pose, the "breeder" is certain to escalate these problems to far more serious proportions. An energy economy based on plutonium-239 means that society will be committed not only to the use of increasingly more accessible nuclear bomb material but also to one of the most lethal elements known to modern science. Plutonium-239 "has been described as 'fiendishly toxic' by some scientists," reports Anthony Ripley. "One of its co-discoverers, Dr. Glen T. Seaborg, former chairman of the [AEC], has said he does not disagree with the description."[34] According to John W. Gofman and Arthur R. Tamplin, two outstanding specialists in nuclear physics and nuclear health problems, the intense alpha radiation produced by the most minute particles of plutonium-239 oxide "in a localized region may be 10 to 1,000 times more effective in producing cancer than would be expected than if the same number of rads were delivered in a more diffuse manner to an organ such as the lung." Gofman and Tamplin estimate that the radionuclide, with a half-life of 24,000 years, can be spread around the earth in such fine particles, "re-suspended in air, and produce lung cancers in generations of humans for 100,000 to 200,000 years."[35] A recent study by the National Resources Defense Council describes plutonium-239 as "one of the most potent cancer producing agents known to man" and demands that the AEC's standards to protect the public from contamination by the element should be 115,000 times more stringent than they are today.[36] A shift from burner to breeder reactors would produce massive quantities of plutonium-239, most of which would doubtless be fissioned as fuel within the reactor core, but substantial quantities of which would unquestionably require storage and seep into the environment. As plutonium-239 and other reactor wastes accumulate, the need to retain strict surveillance of storage depots would extend into future time spans that could only be adequately measured on a geological time scale.

This prospect would be disconcerting enough if current AEC storage practices inspired a reasonable amount of confidence. But recent events have begun to teach us how slovenly, indeed, how grossly irresponsible, the agency has behaved in dealing with more limited and less long-lived wastes than we would expect to accumulate in the next generation or two. According to an astonishing communiqué by the agency released in June 1973, a leak in one of the AEC's Hanford storage tanks near the Columbia River "released 115,000 gallons of highly radioactive (over 500 curies per gallon) liquid into the ground. . . . The most significant radioactive materials in the wastes are strontium-90 with a half-life of 28 years and cesium-137 with a half-life of 30 years." The communiqué adds that a "number of other leaks" have occurred in Hanford since 1958, however, none of this magnitude.[37] In fact, if the earlier leaks are added to the one in June, the total would number in the hundreds of thousands of gallons. The AEC lives on the prayer that the leaked wastes "will be absorbed by the soil and will not reach the ground water 250–300 feet below the tank. However the situation is being carefully monitored since the ground water seeps into the Columbia River seven miles away."[38] One may reasonably ask if the AEC's monitoring is so scrupulous, how could 135,000 gallons have "leaked' 'in the first place.

The frequency and extent to which leaks occur in other storage depots is difficult to judge. But seepages of these wastes into the soil and conceivably into food chains are not always the results of mere "accidents." It taxes one's credulity to learn that the AEC, for the past twenty years, has deliberately disposed of hazardous nuclear wastes by pouring them into open-bottom trenches at the Harford Reservation. These wastes include a cumulative burden of enough plutonium-239 to produce 300 Nagasaki-sized bombs. According to a study made by the agency, one of the trenches accumulated enough plutonium-239 to sustain a nuclear chain reaction that might have spewed radioactive material over wide sectors of the area, with the result that the AEC proposed to remove the plutonium-laden soil from the trench. Yet even while this situation was disclosed to the public, the agency continued to pour radioactive wastes into another trench at a rate of 1.3 million gallons per year.

The growing burden of long-lived global radioactivity with its dire mutagenic and carcinogenic effects; the prospect that the larger this burden, the more incapable humanity may prove of maintaining its surveillance over highly concentrated radioactive wastes in storage depots; the increasing "accidental" seepage of extremely dangerous radioactive materials such as plutonium-239 into the environment—all of these prospects justify a "doomsday syndrome" that Maddox's arts in apologia cannot easily remove, at least from my mind. The "nuclear age," I submit, marks a turning point comparable only to the emergence of life on the planet. For if this "age" means that humanity will be exposed to ever-greater dosages of environmental radiation and if, as seems very likely, future generations will prove incapable of shielding the biosphere from the immense quantities of radioactive wastes that are already slipping from the present generation's control, our species and all advanced organisms will indeed be doomed. The biosphere may be able to recover from the most long-lived chlorinated hydrocarbons known to us; we may restore the integrity of our food supply and the quality of our nutriment by removing hazardous food additives; we and the world of life around us may survive the most terrifying wars with conventional weapons. But we cannot undo the radioactivity that reaches us from the debris of nuclear weapons and the wastes of nuclear plants. Our survival would depend exclusively on the quantity of such wastes to which we are exposed and, ultimately, on the quantity of wastes we accumulate. Like the sand in an hour glass, the extent to which our time is running out is indicated by the number of grains that accumulate. In the case of radioactivity, we cannot reverse the hour glass and start afresh. The grains, in this case, are not symbolic; they are the real thing—the waste material that is accumulating in the radioactive storage tanks, trenches, and reactor cores that are multiplying throughout the world.

I have argued that episodic public efforts to stop the construction of a nuclear plant here or a highway there, valuable as these efforts may be in diminishing the pace of environmental breakdown, will not resolve our fundamental ecological problems. The solution to these problems must be as historic, as fundamental, and as basically social, as the sources of the problems themselves. In contrast to the more apocalyptic voices of my colleagues, I believe we still have the time—the lead time—to make these fundamental changes. I do not believe we have to return to a neolithic technology to do so. Nor do I accept the new "scarcity mentality" that has suddenly been turned on like political tap water by corporate enterprises and the existing administration to counteract the old "affluent mentality" that flowed so fulsomely in the "consumerist" era, when corporations tried to make superprofits by increasing sales rather than raising prices. If anything, we need a new industrial revolution, one which will replace a patently obsolete, highly centralized, wasteful technology designed to produce shabby, short-lived junk commodities in immense quantities by long-lived, high-quality, useful goods that satisfy rational human needs. I do not believe that an ecological philosophy based on renunciation and a labor-intensive, often historically regressive technology is either necessary or socially relevant. Nor do I hold to a "doomsday" mentality that offers us the arrogant option of "first-class passage" on a sinking ship or the well-meaning, if simplistic, scare tactic that we have no more than a decade or so before this planet comes to its well-deserved end. The first leads to an egotistical elitism, even in the fictive death-image it evokes; the second, to passive fatalism.

The real rot lies in the prevailing social order—an order that, by the internal logic of its commodity system and market economy, would devour the entire planet. By this logic, the society would continue to increase its output of garbage even if its population were halved. Its advertising system would be mobilized to sell us three, four, or five color television sets per family instead of one or two. Production rates would continue to soar and the switch turned from "scarcity" to "affluence," or vice versa, depending entirely on the profitability of the commodities that were produced. Pollution would increase and so would waste. *Our Synthetic Environment* is thus, above all, a study in social or "human" ecology, not a pharmacopoeia of chemical products or a psychological study in bad intentions. It does not offer the typically American "happy ending" in which "you," the witless reader, are instructed in the practical details of eluding the snares of greedy, antisocial people of all sorts. Certainly, there is a lot that "you" can do if you happen to live in a reasonably enlightened rural area, if you happen to have access to land that you can garden according to your own principles, and if you are favored with an adequate income to choose the best that you cannot produce for yourself from a rather bad lot. This will not solve all or even most of your environmental problems, and it may consume much of the free time you might otherwise devote to cultivating many of your intellectual interests.

But most people are rooted very much against their wishes in densely populated areas. According to a recent opinion poll, only 13 percent of the people questioned would live in cities if they had a choice, but the opportunity to leave the cities does not exist. Accordingly, they are exposed to polluted air and water; their work is either overly sedentary or exhaustingly muscular. They are compelled to buy processed foods from indifferent retail outlets like supermarkets, and when they seek respite (or catharsis) from the stresses, frustrations, and aggressive impulses generated by their jobs by watching television or going to the movies, they are confronted with violence. The true miracle of our age is that so-called "ordinary people" manage to remain as decent as they are. Indeed, it is testimony to some grandeur in the human spirit that they evince as much kindness, concern, and high-mindedness as they do, for there is absolutely nothing in this society to encourage any humanity or decency in individual behavior.

Our Synthetic Environment is primarily a critical work. It was written to arouse public concern over a relatively new social problem—the problem of environmental breakdown—rather than to provide detailed social solutions. Yet criticism would be thin indeed if it lacked reconstructive guidelines. The book is clearly permeated by a plea for diversity, indeed, a "metaphysics" based on unity in diversity. Diversity is very much in vogue today; twelve years ago it was not. At that time, society was emphasizing the gain in efficiency that accrued from standardization and homogenization.

Perhaps more interestingly, *Our Synthetic Environment* presents ecology not as a narrow scientific discipline but as a broad philosophical and social outlook. I am trying through ecology to heal the wound that was opened by humanity's split with nature thousands of years ago. This theme has been emerging in my own mind as a historic problem that can be resolved only by an ecologically oriented technology, a harmonizing ecological sensibility, and an ecologically oriented society. The point is that it *can* be resolved—the wound *can* be healed— provided one interprets ecology in social, richly utopian terms.

This brings me to the second major theme of this book, namely, decentralization. The closing section of *Our Synthetic Environment* dwells upon the need to overcome the split between town and country, indeed, between mind and body, by decentralizing our cities and restoring the human scale. Apart from nineteenth-century thinkers like Peter Kropotkin and, in our own time, Lewis Mumford, G.E. Gutkind, and Paul Goodman—in short, the libertarian tendency in social thought—this was indeed a novelty for an era that equated centralization with efficiency. As a work on environmental dislocations, the book stood almost alone in emphasizing that a decentralized "community could make maximum use of its own energy resources, such as wind power, solar energy, and hydroelectric power. These sources of energy, so often overlooked because of an almost exclusive reliance on a national division of labor, would help greatly to conserve the remaining supply of high-grade petroleum and coal.

They would almost certainly postpone, if not eliminate, the need for turning to radioactive substances and nuclear reactors as major sources of industrial energy. With more time at his disposal for intensive research, man might learn either to employ solar energy and wind power as the principal sources of energy or eliminate the hazard of radioactive contamination from nuclear reactors."

In 1962, conclusions of this kind, however hesitant they may seem, would have been regarded as preposterously utopian. Today, they have been placed high on the agenda of our most important ecological priorities. I have since elaborated my views on an ecological technology in a large essay, "Toward a Liberatory Technology" (1965), in my book *Post-Scarcity Anarchism* (1971). Yet, in my view, it is not a specific book that has withstood the test of time and retained its relevance after the passing of so many years. What time has verified is a mode of thought— ecological in its natural outlook, libertarian in its social perspectives, and utopian in its ideals. Herein lies the book's reconstructive message. Herein, too, lies the hope, not the shallow optimism, that humanity will find its way, with or without literary works, toward a healing of the ancient split between human and human—and between humanity and nature.

February 1974

Murray Bookchin
School of Human Environment/
School for Metropolitan
and Community Studies
Ramapo College of New Jersey
Mahwah, New Jersey

Social Ecology Studies Program, Goddard College
Plainfield, Vermont

FOOTNOTES TO
COLOPHON EDITION

1. John Osmundsen, "Man Against Nature," *The New York Times Book Review*, May 19, 1963.
2. Ibid.
3. Sigismund Peller, *Cancer in Man* (New York: International Universities Press, Inc., 1952).
4. Leonard Bruckman, "Gasoline Lead Fallout: The Child Poisoner," *The New York Times* (letter to the editor), December 20, 1973.
5. "The FDA's Song-and-Dance on Lead in Canned Milk," *Consumer Reports*, February 1974, p. 106. Consumers Union's account of the FDA's reaction to its research on these lead levels so accurately characterizes the agency's behavior—even as recently as the winter of 1973–74—that it deserves quoting: "When we published our report on high levels of lead in canned evaporated milk last October [*Consumer Reports*], the U.S. Food and Drug Administration went into its now-familiar routine. It pirouetted neatly around our facts, hardly touching them, did a *pas de deux* with the canned-milk trade association, let fly some press releases suggesting our findings were in error and saying that lead had been reduced to acceptable levels in canned milk, and, finally, bowed to the public while applauding itself." I've never known this agency (or the AEC, for that matter) to behave differently. The description is unerring.
6. R.L. Wershaw, "Sources and Behavior of Mercury in Surface Waters" in *Mercury in the Environment* (Washington, D.C.: Government Printing Office, Geological Survey Professional Paper 713, 1970), p. 29.
7. Julian McCaull, "Building a Shorter Life," *Environment*, September 1971, p. 3.
8. Barry Commoner, *The Closing Circle* (New York: Alfred A. Knopf, Inc., 1971), p. 295.
9. Quoted by Gene Marine and Judith Van Allen in *Food Pollution* (New York: Holt, Rinehart and Winston, 1972), p. 69.

10. Quoted by James S. Turner in *The Chemical Feast* (New York: Grossman Publishers, 1970), p. 5.
11. Samuel B. Beaser, "Pancreas and Insulin" in Victor A. Brill, ed., *Pharmacology in Medicine*, 2d ed. (New York: McGraw-Hill Book Co., Inc., 1958), p. 1051.
12. Ibid.
13. Quoted by Turner, *Chemical Feast*, p. 6.
14. Ibid.
15. Ibid.
16. Ibid., p. 13.
17. Ibid.
18. Ibid., p. 14.
19. Ibid., p. 16.
20. Ibid., p. 15.
21. Quoted by Daniel Zwerdling. "Death for Dinner," *The New York Review of Books*, February 21, 1974, p. 22.
22. Ibid.
23. Ibid.
24. Lawrence K. Altman, "Study Finds Americans Exposed to Excessive Monoxide Levels," *The New York Times*, December 20, 1973.
25. Gladwin Hill, "Impure Tapwater a Growing Hazard to the Health of Millions Across U.S.," *The New York Times*, May 13, 1973.
26. Quoted ibid.
27. Thomas Detwyler, *Man's Impact on Environment* (New York: McGraw-Hill Book Co., 1971), p. 429.
28. Max Blumer, "Oil Pollution of the Oceans" in *Oil on the Sea*, David P. Ouet, ed. (New York: Plenum Press, 1969), p. 4.
29. Ibid.
30. John Maddox, *The Doomsday Syndrome* (New York: McGraw-Hill Book Co., 1972). That I find the title of Maddox's book rather fetching does not mean that I think very highly of many of his views. His smugness—a smugness that often verges on apologia—is perhaps more disquieting than some of the exaggerations he imputes to the more "apocalyptic" environmentalists.
31. Quoted in Ralph Lapp, "Nuclear Salvation or Nuclear Folly?" *The New York Times Magazine*, February 10, 1974, p. 69.
32. Ibid., p. 64.
33. Thomas Ehrich, "Atomic Lemons," *The Wall Street Journal*, May 3, 1973.
34. Anthony Ripley, "Law Group Calls for Far Stricter Safeguards on Radiation from Plutonium," *The New York Times*, February 17, 1974.

35. John W. Gofman and Arthur R. Tamplin, *Poisoned Power* (Emmaus, Pa.: Rodale Press, Inc., 1971), p. 61.
36. Ripley, "Law Group Calls for Stricter Safeguards."
37. Event Information Report: 1: 13 June 1973/1654, *Smithsonian Institution, Center for Short-Lived Phenomenon*. This report is reproduced in full in *Alternative Sources of Energy*, July, 1973, p. 50, with a devastating comparison of the soporific press release issued by the AEC on the leakage.
38. Ibid.

Our Synthetic Environment

N O T E

Notes that are principally of bibliographical or scholarly interest have been placed in a separate section at the end of the book.

CHAPTER ONE

The Problem

OUR CHANGED ENVIRONMENT

LIFE in the United States has changed so radically over the past one hundred years that the most wearisome historians tend to become rhapsodic when they describe the new advances that have been made in technology, science, and medicine. We are usually told that early in the last century most Americans lived heroic but narrow lives, eking out a material existence that was insecure and controlled by seasonal changes, drought, and the natural fertility of the soil. Daily work chores were extremely arduous; knowledge, beleaguered by superstition, was relatively crude. Historians with an interest in science often point out that medical remedies were primitive, if not useless; they may have sufficed to relieve the symptoms of common diseases, but they seldom effected a cure. Life was hard and precarious, afflicted by many tragedies that can easily be avoided today.

In contrast with the men of the last century, men today, we are told, have developed nearly complete control over the natural forces that once were the masters of their ancestors. Advances in communication have brought knowledge and safety to the most isolated communities. The most arduous work has now been taken over by machines, and material existence has become secure, even affluent. Common illnesses that once claimed the lives of millions are now easily controlled by a scientific knowledge of disease, effective drugs, new diagnostic devices, and highly developed surgical techniques. The American people, it is claimed, enjoy more leisure, better health, greater longevity, and more varied and abundant diets than did their forebears a hundred years ago.

On the face of it, these statements are true, but by no means are all the advances as beneficial as the historians would have us believe. Recent changes in our synthetic environment have created new problems that are as numerous as those which burdened the men of the past. For example, soon nearly 70 per cent of the American population will be living in large metropolitan centers, such as New York, Chicago, and Los Angeles. They will be exposed in ever-greater numbers to automobile exhausts and urban air pollutants. Perhaps an even larger percentage of the employed population will be working in factories and offices. These people will be deprived of sunlight and fresh air during the best hours of the day. Factory and office work, while less arduous than in the past, is becoming more intensive. Although the working day early in the last century was very long, "the worker worked comparatively slowly, and both the employer and employee gave relatively little thought to productivity." Today, employers require a greater output per hour from each worker. The use of machines tends to make work monotonous and sedentary, often exhausting human nerves as completely as manual work exhausted human muscles. Modern man is far less physically active than his forebears were. He observes rather than performs, and uses less and less of his body at work and play. His diet, although more abundant, consists of highly processed foods. These foods contain a disconcertingly large amount of pesticide residues, coloring and flavoring matter, preservatives, and chemical "technological aids," many of which may impair his health. His waterways and the air he breathes contain not only the toxic wastes of the more familiar industries but radioactive pollutants, the byproducts of peacetime uses of nuclear energy and nuclear weapons tests.

With the rise of these problems, dramatic changes have occurred in the incidence of disease. In 1900, infectious diseases, such as pneumonia, influenza, and tuberculosis, were the principal causes of death. Death from heart disease and cancer occupied a secondary place in American vital statistics. Fifty years later, mortality rates from infectious diseases had declined to a fraction of what they had been, but the percentage of deaths from heart disease and malignant tumors had more than doubled. It is very difficult to obtain reliable comparative statistics on the incidence of chronic, or persistent, diseases, but we can regard it as almost certain that the proportion of chronically ill individuals in the American population has increased. In any case, millions of Americans today suffer from major chronic disorders. Nearly 5 million people are afflicted with heart disease; another 5 million have high blood pressure. More than 12 million suffer from arthritis, 4 million from asthma, and at least 700,000 from cancer. Additional millions suffer from diabetes, kidney disease, and disorders of the nervous system.

Because many of these illnesses claim the lives of

elderly people, we tend to associate chronic diseases with the aging process, and we usually explain their widespread occurrence by the fact that people are living longer. Men must die of something. With a reduction in the number of deaths from tuberculosis, influenza, and childhood infections, the diseases of aging people, it is claimed, should be expected to dominate our vital statistics. But are these diseases strictly products of the aging process? Do we have any evidence that they arise from basic physical disturbances peculiar to senescence? The answer is almost certainly no. Many disorders which afflict young people are precisely those so-called "degenerative diseases" that physicians and laymen associate with the retrogressive physical changes of old age.

Consider the age distribution in the incidence of cancer. Although many types of cancer are found mostly after the fourth or fifth decade of life, a surprisingly large number of varieties occur most frequently in childhood, youth, and early maturity. Cancers of the kidney and the adrenal glands usually appear before the age of four. Bone cancers reach their highest incidence in the ten-to-twenty-four age group. Malignant tumors of the testes usually occur in infancy and at maturity. So deeply entrenched was the notion that malignant tumors are diseases of elderly people that for many years physicians often discounted early symptoms of certain cancers in children. We now know that cancer in children occurs in nearly all the major physical organs of the body.

Today, cancer is second only to accidents as a leading cause of death in American children over one year of age. Although mortality rates for childhood cancers fluctuate from year to year, they have moved in a decidedly upward direction over the past two decades; for American children under fifteen years of age, they rose 28 per cent between 1940 and 1955. In 1959, cancer claimed 4,100 lives and accounted for 12 per cent of all deaths in children between the ages of one and fourteen. These statistics make it hazardous to say that the illness is essentially part of the aging process. Strong reasons exist for suspecting that environmental factors contribute significantly to increases in death from cancer among young people.

The same suspicions can be extended to heart and vascular disorders. Until recently, heart disease in young people was caused primarily by infectious illnesses. Rheumatic heart disease, following streptococcal infections, claimed the lives of many children between the ages of ten and fourteen. Fortunately, the incidence of rheumatic fever has been reduced dramatically by the use of antibiotics. On the other hand, coronary heart disease was generally regarded as a typical degenerative illness of older people, attributable to the onset of vascular disorders well beyond the peak of life. The disease seemed to be a culmination of the aging process. This view, too, is no longer a deeply entrenched medical opinion. Atherosclerosis, the precursor of coronary heart attacks, is not a universal feature of old age. On autopsy, many an octogenarian has been found to have coronary arteries that a man in his forties would be fortunate to possess.

Even more disconcerting is the unexpectedly high incidence of coronary illness now known to exist among young people. During the Korean War, the U. S. Armed Forces Institute of Pathology performed a series of autopsies on the bodies of 300 American soldiers, most of whom had been killed in front-line areas. Careful attempts were made to exclude cases in which there had been clinical evidence of coronary disease. The investigators, Enos, Holmes, and Beyer, observed that the average age in "200 cases was 22.1 years. The ages in the first 98

cases were not recorded except that the oldest patient
was 33. . . . In 77.3% of the hearts, some gross evidence of coronary atherosclerosis was found."

In at least 12 per cent of the hearts, the obstruction
of one or more major coronary arteries exceeded 50 per
cent of the arterial passageway. These are extremely high
figures for young men who presumably were qualified
for military service. A comparative study performed on
the bodies of 350 Americans in Boston and 352 Japanese
in Fukuoka "disclosed a considerable difference in the
severity of coronary atherosclerosis" between the two
national groups. In the American group every individual
had some degree of atherosclerosis by the second decade
of life, whereas Japanese could be found without the disease in the fifth and sixth decades. Comparing the extent
of the arterial surface involved and the severity of the
lesions found in the two groups, the investigators emphasize that "there was at least a two-decade difference
in the progression of atherosclerosis. The average American of age 40 and the average Japanese of age 60 presented comparable arterial disease."

In all probability, data of this sort merely supply us
with fragmentary evidence of the extent to which chronic
and degenerative illnesses are invading the younger age
groups of our population. Many individuals seem to be
succumbing to degenerative diseases long before they
reach the prime of life. Not only is cancer a leading cause
of death in childhood and youth, but the results obtained
by Enos and his co-workers suggest that many American
males between twenty and thirty years of age are on the
brink of major cardiac disease. Although most of these
individuals are likely to exhibit no clinical symptoms of
vascular disorders—indeed, they would probably be regarded as healthy in routine medical examinations—it is
reasonable to say that they are ill. If diseases of this kind

represent the normal deterioration of the body, then human biology is taking a patently abnormal turn. A large number of people are breaking down prematurely.

Heredity, of course, may "play a role"—to use a well-worn qualification. But medical history warns us that genetic explanations of disease, particularly common diseases that afflict large sections of the population, are often a refuge for incomplete knowledge. Many such explanations are being contradicted by research. For example, it is very doubtful whether the "inherently" weak and sick, who presumably were rescued by modern medicine from the fatal infections of the past, are destined to be victims of cancer. In fact, there is good reason to believe that the body's mechanisms for resistance to cancers are entirely distinct from those that combat infections.* "The old idea that chronic diseases are 'degenerative,' or inevitable concomitants of aging," observes Lester Breslow, of the California State Department of Public Health, "is giving way to the modern idea that the origins of chronic disease lie in specific external causes which can be discovered and thus controlled." With all due respect to genetics and to theories that attribute chronic disease to senescence, it would be more rewarding to examine the changes that have occurred over the past half century in man's diet, habits, forms of work, and physical surroundings.

* Terminal cancer patients, whose initial resistance to experimental inoculations of cancer cells is virtually nil, may nevertheless offer marked resistance to harmful bacteria and viruses. A team of Sloan-Kettering researchers inoculated fifteen terminal cancer patients with live cancer cells and germs. Thirteen patients showed no resistance to the cells, which took root and formed vigorous cancers. This will not ordinarily occur in individuals who do not have cancer. But the same cancer patients produced effective antibodies against inoculations of disease-causing bacteria and viruses.

ENVIRONMENT AND ILLNESS

A BALANCED ATTITUDE toward environmentally induced illness has generally been the exception rather than the rule. In the past, as medical fashions changed, opinion would tend to swing from one oversimplification to another. For a long time, the germ theory of disease discouraged giving serious attention to the environment as a major factor in illness. Attempts to investigate the relationship between environmental change and disease were viewed as a regression to the pre-Pasteur days of medicine. The goals of research, it was declared, are to discover and destroy the microorganisms that cause illness. The physician was conceived to be locked in a struggle with microbes, and the human organism was regarded as virtually the only legitimate arena for waging this conflict. The synthetic and social environments outside man's body seemed irrelevant to the basic problems of diagnosis and therapy, except where sanitation and the isolation of individuals with communicable diseases were involved.*

This view has never fully explained society's experience with tuberculosis. In Europe, tuberculosis had always flourished among the urban poor, but except for occasional flare-ups here and there, the disease had never

---

* In a brilliant survey of this period, Iago Galdston observes that as late as the 1920's "few among the medical leaders gave much consideration (other than isolation, sterilization) to the 'conditions of person and environment' that favored the agents of infection. The attitude of the medical profession and of the public health workers was well reflected in the campaign slogans forecasting the stamping out of this or that infectious disease by the end of some ten, fifteen, or twenty years. The talk was of war, and the enemy was the tubercle bacillus, the gonococcus, the spirochete!"

assumed the epidemic proportions of cholera and typhus. With the Industrial Revolution, however, tuberculosis became especially widespread and virulent. The crowding of uprooted rural folk into cities, the impoverishment and overcrowding of the new industrial laboring classes, and the decline in nearly all standards of nutrition, health, and sanitation raised tuberculosis from a tenacious but controlled urban disease to an illness pandemic throughout the Western world. The disease did not begin to recede until sweeping reforms were made in the economic life of Europe and America. It was brought under control only after the working classes had achieved shorter working hours, higher income, better housing, and improved sanitation—in short, after the standard of living had been raised. It is no overstatement to declare that the social reformers who were instrumental in getting children removed from the factories and helped bring about higher wages and the eight-hour working day did more to control tuberculosis than did Koch, who discovered the tubercle bacillus.

When it became evident that the incidence of tuberculosis could be attributed to social factors as well as to the presence of a germ, another oversimplification took hold in medical circles. The disease was transformed into a model of environmentally induced illness. In respiratory tuberculosis, a simple, dramatic interaction seems to exist between an infectious agent and environmental conditions. On the one hand, without the tubercle bacillus there can be no tuberculosis; the germ is a disease-causing, or pathogenic, agent. On the other hand, many healthy people in Europe and the United States have had arrested cases of tuberculosis without ever knowing it. The bacillus may continue to exist in an individual's body with no noticeable impairment of the lungs or occurrence of the illness. In most cases, the germ becomes harmful only when physical resistance is lowered. All the elements in the relationship between the illness and the environment seem to be easily determined. A known and observable microorganism can be isolated from the sputum of all tubercular patients. The environmental changes that foster tuberculosis, such as a deterioration in diet and working conditions, can be interpreted in terms of calories, minerals, vitamins, and even working hours. Normally the disease can be arrested by sufficient quantities of nourishing foods, by rest, and by the administration of drugs.

In contrast with tuberculosis, however, the specific causes of many chronic and degenerative diseases are very obscure. Illness may occur under "favorable" as well as "unfavorable" environmental conditions. Heart disease, cancer, arthritis, and diabetes—the most important degenerative diseases of our time—claim their victims from the well-to-do and poor alike. The environmental conditions that encourage infectious disorders, such as poverty and arduous work, are often absent from the lives of persons afflicted with a degenerative disease. The course taken by a degenerative illness is highly complex, varying markedly from individual to individual. The relationship between environmental change and degenerative disorders lacks the simplicity and drama encountered in cases of tuberculosis. Hence, any emphasis on environmental change in the study of heart disease, cancer, and similar illnesses still meets with a certain amount of reserve and distrust. Everything seems to be ambiguous—the environment, its relationship to the disease, and, at times, even the disease itself.

But the picture is not so bleak as it seems. An illness is obviously environmentally induced when it becomes widespread following a major environmental change.

Sharp differences of opinion are likely to arise when the change conflicts with an entrenched point of view in a particular medical specialty. A specialist in tuberculosis, for example, will regard an environmental change as harmful when it results in a reduced consumption of food and in increased physical activity. Many specialists in heart disorders, however, will regard the same change as beneficial. The traditional image of a healthy man—a plump and relatively inactive individual with a hearty appetite—was created in the last century, when tuberculosis was by far the major disease. The new, emerging image of a healthy individual is represented by a lean man who eats sparingly and who engages in a great deal of physical activity. At first glance, we seem to encounter a sharp conflict of views over the factors that promote or inhibit environmentally induced illnesses. But on closer inspection it becomes evident that both views have a common point of departure, namely, in immoderate prescriptions for diet, work, and play. From the extremes of malnutrition and arduous labor, the environmental pendulum in the Western world has begun to swing to the extremes of overnourishment and physical inactivity.

Let us examine some of the dietary extremes. At the turn of the century, many Americans ate too little to meet their physical needs. Today, they eat too much. Although the average caloric intake may be falling, the decline in the need for food is moving at a faster rate than the decline in the intake of food. A farm laborer requires about four thousand calories a day to maintain good health. Engaged in light office work, the same man would seldom require more than two thousand calories daily. Yet it is doubtful whether most Americans engaged in sedentary work limit themselves to so modest an intake of food. They tend to overeat in relation to the work they do. In fact, the average American male over thirty years of age weighs about ten to fifteen pounds more than he should.

Not only does he overeat, but he eats too much of the wrong foods. The annual per capita consumption of sugar, for example, has increased enormously in the past fifty years. "Including sugar consumed in candies, sirups, jams, and jellies, as well as for table use and in cooking," observes L. Jean Bogert, "sugar consumption in the United States amounts to over 100 pounds per person yearly, or about a half pound each day for every person in the country. Our annual candy bill is over a billion dollars and has increased over 1000 per cent in the last 60 years." There has been no noteworthy decline in the over-all intake of fats. Although the consumption of butter has fallen off, the per capita intake of margarine and hydrogenated oils has increased.

Has this new form of an old environmental excess played any role in creating the modern disease landscape? The answer is almost assuredly yes. Obesity is closely linked with diabetes. Although a predisposition to diabetes is hereditary, the disease occurs primarily in overweight individuals. Proper management of the disorder involves weight regulation as well as dietary control and the use of insulin. Surprisingly, there also seems to be strong statistical evidence that obese individuals are more disposed to cancer than those who maintain their proper weight. The evidence has been summarized in a popular work on nutrition by Norman Jolliffe, of the New York City Department of Health. "Life insurance figures show that of all men who bought their policies at age 45 or over, a 25 per cent higher death rate from cancer is noted in that portion of the group which is 15 per cent or more overweight. Overweight women have a 30 to 45 per cent greater chance of developing a cancer of the uterus than those who are not fat. There is also evidence from the experimental laboratory that normal weight mice are less susceptible to both spontaneous and induced tumor formations than fat ones."

A strong suspicion exists that diets high in dairy fats, animal fats, and hydrogenated oils are implicated in the rising incidence of coronary heart disease. During World War II, the reduction in the amount of fatty goods in the diets of the people in German-occupied countries was followed by a sharp decline in the number of deaths from coronary heart illness. When the occupation came to an end and animal fats returned to the diet, the coronary death rate rose dramatically. The data collected from occupied Europe led to studies of the eating habits of Bantu and whites in South Africa, native and Hawaiian Japanese, Trappist and Benedictine monks, and many other related communities where the effects of low- and high-fat diets could be compared in a meaningful way. The Bantu, the native Japanese, and the Trappists, who consume very small quantities of meat and dairy foods, are not seriously burdened by coronary heart illness. Their counterparts, whose diets are rich in fatty foods, have a high incidence of the disease. It has been established by many researchers that the consumption of animal fats raises the level of cholesterol in the blood. The greater the amount of cholesterol deposited in the coronary arteries, the greater the chances of a coronary heart attack. It should be emphasized that the level of cholesterol in the blood can be raised by non-dietary as well as dietary factors and that high cholesterol levels do not necessarily result in vascular disorders. Nevertheless, there is strong statistical support for the belief that the high levels of cholesterol in the blood produced by a normally fatty diet contribute to the rising incidence of coronary heart illness.

These illustrations, needless to say, do not argue for the German occupation of Europe, the Bantu diet, or the virtues of monastic life among the Trappists. The Bantu diet is seriously deficient in nutrients vital to the maintenance of good health, and Trappist monks, in contrast with the Benedictines, engage in a great deal of physical work. Many questions could be raised about non-dietary factors that may tip the scales for or against a high incidence of coronary heart illness. What role do certain undesirable habits, such as cigarette smoking, play in the occurrence of the disease? Is coronary heart illness promoted by physical inactivity and obesity, as some authorities have suggested? Indeed, does any single environmental factor determine the incidence of vascular and heart disorders in a given community? Whatever may prove to be the relationship between these diseases and diet, other factors are suspected of contributing to their occurrence, notably stress, sedentary forms of work, smoking, and a poor genetic endowment.

The problems of research would be simplified immeasurably if every environmental factor that plays a role in degenerative illnesses could be isolated and its effects subjected to precise analysis. Such clear-cut results are likely to be the exception rather than the rule. More than may be suggested by comparative studies of diet, the importance of any factor in chronic and degenerative diseases varies from individual to individual, from region to region, and from illness to illness. In the case of cigarette smoking, for example, the amount of nicotine, tars, and other harmful substances taken in varies with the brand of cigarette, the quantity of cigarettes consumed, and the amount of each cigarette that is smoked. Some individuals may have a stronger reaction to a given intake of nicotine than others. Those who exhibit no apparent ill effects from the long-term intake of nicotine may respond very gravely to tobacco tars. Finally, in many individuals smoking may tip the scales in favor of degenerative diseases that are basically caused by a harmful diet, air pollution, and stress. The analyst is confronted with a constellation of factors in which each factor is meaningful only in relation to all the others.

And here a typical disagreement arises. In the absence of conclusive evidence that a single factor contributes to all cases of an illness, many researchers are inclined to distrust the constellation as a whole. Complexity is regarded as "ambiguity," and the relationship between environment and degenerative illnesses is dismissed as "vague." This kind of thinking is characteristic of our modern *Weltgeist.* "We prefer to study systems that can easily be isolated and approached by simple methods," observed Alexis Carrel more than twenty years ago. "We generally neglect the more complex. Our mind has a partiality for precise and definitive solutions and for the resulting intellectual security. We have an almost irresistible tendency to select the subjects of our investigations for their technical facility and clearness rather than for their importance. Thus, modern physiologists principally concern themselves with physico-chemical phenomena taking place in living animals, and pay less attention to physiological and functional processes. The same thing happens with physicians when they specialize in subjects whose techniques are easy and already known rather than in degenerative diseases, neuroses, and psychoses, whose study would require the use of imagination and the creation of new methods."

This comment is still valid today, especially as it applies to attitudes toward complex, environmentally induced illnesses. The study of chronic and degenerative disorders still calls for imaginative departures from conventional approaches to disease. Tuberculosis can be explained by a germ and a number of clear-cut environmental factors. No such explanation can be found for many chronic and degenerative illnesses. Where a contributory factor, such as tobacco tars or a high intake of fatty foods, is evident in the occurrence of a disease, it may prove to be just one of many causes. Moreover, whereas a germ has its own fixed natural history, the factors that promote degenerative illnesses often originate in man's rapidly changing synthetic environment. The influence of environmental factors, in turn, can be seen only through the human organism, whose individual differences often make it difficult to achieve clear-cut analyses.

But as research progresses, the role of environmental change in forming the modern disease landscape emerges more clearly. Many physicians are now convinced that cigarette smoking, obesity, stress, and a fatty diet have contributed significantly to the high incidence of atherosclerosis and cancer. The link between environment and illness is becoming difficult to ignore. This is not to say that every degenerative disease is environmentally induced. But it is becoming evident that all the revolutionary changes in our synthetic environment, from the rise of an urban society to the use of nuclear energy, have profound biological implications, and that these changes have added an environmental dimension to nearly every area of public health.

THE HUMAN BODY AND ILLNESS

THE EFFECT of our synthetic environment on health is difficult to gauge for still another reason; namely, the rigid, rather schematic approach to illness that generally prevails today. What, it may be asked, is disease? Or to put the question another way: At what point does a healthy individual become ill? These questions are not easy to answer. But the difficulties involved deserve careful examination, for they are closely related to the problems created by environmentally induced disease.

Many physicians tend to approach the human organism with a fixed threshold of illness in mind. On one side of the threshold, the body is conceived as being in good health; on the other side, it is diseased and requires treatment. The line between health and disease is generally drawn as sharply as possible. The body ordinarily must reach a certain degree of disequilibrium and damage before it is regarded as ill. This approach would be excusable if it could be attributed merely to a fragmentary knowledge of the complex processes that take place in the human body. But the approach is due, in no small measure, to a lack of interest in the "healthy" side of the threshold, where the conditions for illness are slowly created by insidious changes in the organism. Ignorance is perpetuated by a complacent indifference to many of the basic problems involved in the transition from health to disease.

The validity of this schematic approach has been challenged repeatedly by the findings of modern research in biochemistry, particularly by the results obtained from studies of human cells. It should be a truism that the majority of human illnesses are fought out on the cellular, even the molecular, level of life. Whether we survive an illness or not depends on the number and types of cells that are damaged during the course of the disease. Ordinarily, however, we tend to regard the damaged tissues of the body as the passive victims of physical disorders. When infections occur, we think of white blood cells rushing to devour bacteria and of antibodies inhibiting the effects of toxins. We seem to believe that resistance to disease is exclusively the function of certain specialized organs and systems within the body. The health and resistance of cells that are involved in the more routine functions of an organism are seldom regarded as important in the prevention or outcome of an illness.

Yet many human disorders would be difficult to explain without acknowledging the significance of general cellular well-being. An example is supplied by pellagra. Pellagra is caused by a deficiency of niacin, a member of the vitamin-B complex. A lack of niacin or of the amino acid tryptophan (a chemical precursor of niacin) produces a broad spectrum of disorders, ranging from skin eruptions to mental aberrations. As the disease progresses, changes occur in the tissues of the mouth, followed by ulcerations, a slough of dead cells, and the proliferation of disease-causing germs. At this stage, secondary infections, such as trench mouth, often set in. The infections are caused primarily, not by the germs, many of which are present in healthy individuals, but rather by molecular changes within the cells which slowly lower the defenses of tissues in the mouth. The cells that line the mouth and tongue are in ill health. To borrow the words of a great American nutritionist, they have suffered a loss of "tissue integrity." The decline in cellular health, often very protracted and insidious, may not be clinically perceptible for a long time.

The concept that cells can be in ill health long before the appearance of symptoms in the form of a conventional disease, receives strong support from cancer.*

---

* Cancer cells can be regarded as ill not only because they are abnormal and produce disorders in the organism as a whole, but also because their biochemical processes seem to be impaired. For example, Otto Warburg, of the Max Planck Institute for Cell Physiology in Berlin, has advanced the theory that cancer is due to

Many functional differences distinguish cancerous from non-cancerous cells. Cancer cells not only multiply uncontrollably at a given site; in many cases they also spread, or metastasize, to vital organs elsewhere in the body. Metastasis accounts for most of the lives claimed by the disease. Normal cells multiply in a regulated manner and, except for certain highly specialized cells, never migrate from the tissues in which they originate. Careful studies of the development of cancer in experimental animals suggest that cells seldom become malignant until they have passed through many gradations of ill health. Any meaningful discussion of the disease must take account of healthy cells, cells in varying degrees of ill health, pre-cancerous cells, which impart abnormal characteristics to tissues, and finally true cancer cells, which reproduce uncontrollably. Few if any of these gradations are likely to manifest themselves in noticeable symptoms of disease. Although the transition from normal to pre-cancerous and cancerous cells may occur very rapidly, it is highly probable that the majority of malignant tumors arise only after a cell and its descendants have silently traveled a long road from health to a pre-cancerous and then a cancerous state.

That this kind of deterioration can occur should not surprise us. Cellular metabolism is so complex that many things can go wrong in a cell without producing major symptoms of disease in the organism as a whole. A living cell engages in an enormous variety of chemical operations in which extremely complex molecules are built up and broken down at a rapid pace. A delicate balance

changes in the manner in which cells obtain energy. According to Warburg, cancer-causing substances damage the cell's respiratory mechanisms, causing it to obtain energy by fermentation. In cases in which cancer is caused by viruses, the cells can be regarded as infected; their reproductive apparatus is controlled or deranged by the presence of an alien agent.

exists between the absorption of nutrients and the excretion of waste products. If this balance is altered a trifle for any length of time, dysfunctions will occur in the cell. If it is altered a bit more, vague symptoms of illness may appear. If blood or oxygen is denied to certain organs of the body for a very short period of time, irreparable, even fatal, damage will occur.

But many disorders may persist without ever assuming an overt form. The activities of cells, tissues, and organs may be retarded; adverse changes may occur in the body's complex metabolic functions; in time, physical activity may be impaired and longevity reduced. If changes of this nature occur in a large number of individuals, our standards of public health may be lowered imperceptibly. Such individuals will not be regarded as ill in the conventional sense of the term. In fact, until they are afflicted with cancer or heart attacks, they will satisfy all the schematic criteria for glowing health.

Fortunately, the need to give greater attention to covert, or subclinical, disturbances in the human body is gaining increasing recognition. For example, it is worth noting the way in which former U. S. Surgeon General Leroy E. Burney discusses the hazards that are created by low-level concentrations of chemical toxicants in water. "They are not killing us or making us clinically ill. But how does the human body react to steady doses of diluted chemicals? What happens if the concentration increases, either suddenly or gradually? We cannot say that we know the answers." The same problem is raised by Robert A. Kehoe, of the University of Cincinnati. After a review of the toxicants, physical hazards, radioactive pollutants, and "welter of activities" created by our synthetic environment, Kehoe asks: "But what are the consequences, through the working life time, of the frequent, almost daily, impacts of individual and collective insults of minor or sub-clinical severity?" Attention should be focused on Burney and Kehoe's concern for subclinical damage, a concept that is not particularly congenial to the outlook of the American medical community.

It is difficult to see how the problem of subclinical damage can be ignored in investigations of cancer and nutritional disorders. Researchers are constantly seeking better methods for the early diagnosis of malignant and pre-malignant tumors. But diagnostic techniques, however desirable, are not at issue here. If it can be inferred from the complexity of man's metabolism that ill health can exist long before it becomes medically evident, it follows that the greatest care should be exercised in changing man's environment. Where changes are desirable, they should be preceded by meticulous and imaginative studies. And where changes are necessary, every precaution should be taken to minimize any ill effects they may have on the human body. It would be utter folly to introduce needless changes in man's diet, forms of work, habits, and physical surroundings without investigating their effects from the broadest perspective of public health.

Environmental changes should be studied not only in relation to the more dramatic effects they have on man; study should also be focused on the subtle changes produced in tissues and bodily functions. In addition research should be directed toward disorders that may arise years after a new product is offered for public consumption. Whenever an inessential product is suspected of being harmful to man, its sale or distribution should be prohibited. The concept of environmentally induced illness should include all structural levels of the human organism and encompass not only present but also future generations.

MAN AND THE NATURAL WORLD

UNFORTUNATELY, the amount of research devoted to environmental health falls far short of current needs. Many important problems are being neglected for want of funds and trained personnel. Where research is intensive, it is often fragmentary and un-co-ordinated. "Separate approaches to specific problems have had great practical value," notes a recent report by the Surgeon General to the House Appropriations Committee. "They have provided effective mechanisms for getting at critical phases of important problems. . . . But the many and complex interrelationships among those problems have become increasingly apparent, and it is obvious that they must be considered as parts of a whole. . . . To achieve a 'total view,' there must be an integration of research and control methods. The knowledge and skills of many professional specialties—physicians, engineers, physicists, chemists, educators, statisticians among them—must be further coordinated in seeking scientifically sound answers to the many challenging questions in the field of environmental health."

These words are more a complaint against the absence of a "total view" than a tribute to "separate approaches to specific problems." Time is running out. Many passages in the Surgeon General's report would be dismissed as doleful exaggerations if we were not aware of the fact that they come from an official and highly responsible source. "New chemicals, many of them with toxic properties or capabilities, are being produced and marketed, and put into use at a rapid rate," the report observes. "These include plastics, plasticizers, additives to fuels and foods, pesticides, detergents, abrasives." An estimated "400-500 totally new chemicals are put into use each year. . . . Although many commonly used chemicals are checked for toxicity, much is still unknown about their long-term potential hazards." The report warns that while "the modern supermarket and frozen food locker permit the use of a wide variety of foods, with resulting nutritional benefits, . . . modern methods of growing and processing foods introduce new hazards of pesticide spray residues, preservatives and other food additives, and even contaminants related to packaging, which require attention for control." An ominous generalization at the beginning of the report could well serve for its conclusion: "It is not being overdramatic to suggest that threats from our environment, actual and potential, can not only generate wholly undesirable effects on the health and well-being of isolated individuals, but under certain circumstances could affect large segments of our population and conceivably threaten the very existence of our Nation."

Despite the frankness of the Surgeon General's report, the federal government not only has failed to meet these problems resolutely but has directly and indirectly contributed to them. The indirect contribution was made through inaction. It took nearly a half century of debate, both in and out of Congress, to obtain national legislation which made manufacturers legally responsible for pre-testing food additives. Until 1959 the job of establishing whether a food additive was harmful was performed by the Food and Drug Administration, and attempts to prohibit the use of such additives often involved long and costly judicial proceedings. The same legislative procrastination is now being encountered in connection with new environmental health problems. Although air and water pollution has reached staggering proportions, national legislation to combat it is creeping forward at a snail's pace. At the same time, government-subsidized nuclear energy programs are creating one of the most hazardous sources of air and water pollution in man's environment. The harmful consequences of these programs outweigh any improvements that may have resulted from recent laws to control food additives. On balance, the over-all situation is deteriorating with every passing year.

The problems of our synthetic environment can be summed up by saying that nonhuman interests are superseding many of our responsibilities to human biological welfare. To a large extent, man is no longer working for himself. Many fields of knowledge and many practical endeavors that were once oriented toward the satisfaction of basic human wants have become ends in themselves, and to an ever-greater degree these new ends are conflicting with the requirements for human health. The needs of industrial plants are being placed before man's need for clean air; the disposal of industrial wastes has gained priority over the community's need for clean water. The most pernicious laws of the market place are given precedence over the most compelling laws of biology.

Understandably, a large number of people have reacted to the nonhuman character of our synthetic environment by venerating nature as the only source of health and well-being. The natural state, almost without reservation, is regarded as preferable to the works of modern man and the environment he has created for himself. The term "natural" tends to become synonymous with "primitive." The more man's situation approximates that of his primitive forebears, it is thought, the more he will be nourished by certain quasi-mystical wellsprings of health and virtue. In view of the mounting problems created by our synthetic environment, this renunciation of science and technology—indeed, of civilization—would be almost tempting if it were not manifestly impractical. An unqualified idealization of the natural world involves an acceptance of many environmental conditions that are distinctly unfavorable to human life. Until the advent of civilization, nature shaped the course of human evolution with severity, visiting death on all individuals who could not satisfy her rigorous requirements for survival. Millions of people are living today who could not have met the demands of a more primitive way of life. They would have perished on the battlegrounds of natural selection as surely as the young and fit are now destroyed on the battlegrounds of modern war.

A much greater impediment to a rational outlook, however, springs from a tendency to ignore man's dependence on the natural world. The extent of this dependence cannot be emphasized too strongly. The great diversity of racial types reminds us that human communities have followed their own distinctive lines of evolution. Each has adapted itself over many millennia to different climatic and physical conditions. Many subtle differences in needs exist among human groups, indeed among individual types. "Changing conditions of life affect individuals and groups," observed Wade H. Brown, of the Rockefeller Institute, a generation ago, "but as individuals differ in respect of their inherent constitutional equipment, they differ also in their reactions to influences of all kinds. Some are capable of immediate and complete adjustment, others are slow to respond or are incapable of adjustment, so that when members of a group are subjected to a change in the conditions of life or are exposed to infection under favorable or unfavorable conditions, the response obtained varies according to the capacities of the individual." Medicine and technology are providing only partial compensation for the harmful effects of new diets, changed modes of work, and unfamiliar climates. Technicians can supply a fair-skinned man with air conditioning in hot tropical regions. They can clothe a Negro in effective heat-retaining garments in the cold northlands. But these measures are only *ad hoc* solutions to the threat of extinction. In their new environment, both men must function as limited individuals, restricting their activities and normal mode of life.

At the same time, we should not lose sight of the needs all men have in common. Every human being has minimum requirements for certain nutrients. Although human diets may be modified by differences in climate, work, and available foods, these modifications usually represent differences in nutritional emphasis, whether on proteins, carbohydrates, or fats. The human body must be employed in a variety of physical activities, or it will weaken and health and possibly longevity will be adversely affected. New toxicants dangerous to men of one race are equally hazardous to men of other races. The appearance of these toxic agents in the atmosphere, water, and foods threatens the health of every human being. As we shall see later, the extent to which they threaten man may differ appreciably from the extent to which they threaten other species, so that experimental work with animals does not always disclose the damage the new toxicants produce in human beings. For the present, it should be emphasized that the limits of environmental change were staked out by forces well beyond human control. After aeons of biological evolution, man is subject to unrelenting anatomical and physiological demands. If these demands are ignored, he faces the revenge of his own body in the form of early debilitation and a shortened life span. His basic needs for optimal health have largely been decided for him by his long development as a unique animal organism.

Lastly, man must live in harmony with myriad forms of plants and animals, many of which are indispensable to his survival. In the long run, a fertile soil is just as important for human health as clean air and water. Adequately nourished animals are as necessary for man's well-being as adequately nourished human tissues. Any serious disorders in the land or in plants and animals eventually produce disorders in the human body. Man tends to weaken and give way to illness as the natural preconditions for his health are undermined by erosion, disease, or pollution. Nearly all the abuses he inflicts on soil, plants, and animals are returned to him in kind, perhaps indirectly, but all the more malignantly because the damage is often far advanced before it can be seen and corrected.

We tend to view problems in the world of living things—the biosphere—with the same schematic approach that we bring to environmental health problems. We demand evidence of a marked injury to man's natural surroundings before we are ready to agree that there exist problems that require solutions. We make sharp distinctions between order and disorder in nature, just as we draw a sharp line between health and disease in man. Nevertheless, the same kinds of qualitative problems we encounter in the physiology of human beings reappear in ecology; that is, in the study of how living things interact with one another and with their environment. Every organism has its own environmentally induced illnesses. The environmentally induced diseases of plants and animals, like the chronic and degenerative diseases of man, are due to a multiplicity of factors. And just as many disorders may persist in man without ever assuming an overt form, covert illness may persist in plants and animals without ever producing clear-cut symptoms of disease.

The caution that should be exercised in changing our synthetic environment should also be exercised in changing the biosphere. Never before in man's history has there been a greater need for what Ralph and Mildred Buchsbaum call the "ecological viewpoint" toward man's influence on the natural world. This viewpoint is "the conservative view of man's relation to his total environment. It holds that an environmental setting developed by natural selection over many millions of years must be considered to have some merit. Anything so complicated as a planet inhabited by more than a million and a half species of plants and animals, all of them living together in a more or less balanced equilibrium in which they continually use and reuse the same molecules of the soil and air, cannot be improved by aimless and uninformed tinkering. All changes in a complex mechanism involve some risk and should be undertaken only after careful study of all the facts available. Changes should be made on a small scale first so as to provide a test before they are widely applied. When information is incomplete, changes should stay close to the natural processes which have in their favor the indisputable evidence of having supported life for a very long time."

CHAPTER TWO

Agriculture and Health

SOIL AND AGRICULTURE

PROBLEMS of soil and agriculture seldom arouse the interest of urban dwellers. Town and country have become so sharply polarized that the city man and the farmer live in widely separated, contrasting, and often socially antagonistic worlds. The average resident of an American metropolis knows as little about the problems of growing food as the average farmer knows about the problems of mass transportation. The city man, to be sure, does not need to be reminded that good soil is important for successful farming. He recognizes the necessity for conservation and careful management of the land. But his knowledge of food cultivation—its techniques, problems, and prospects—is limited. He leaves the land in trust to the farmer in the belief that modern agricultural methods cannot fail to produce attractive and nourishing food.

In reality, however, modern agronomy is beset with highly controversial problems, many of which deeply concern the welfare of urban man. It has been vehemently argued and as vigorously denied that soil fertility has a profound influence on the quality of food. According to some agronomists, deterioration in the fertility and structure of the soil results in nutritionally inferior crops. Such crops may satisfy the demands of hunger but not necessarily the requirements of human physiology. If a shift from high- to low-quality crops occurs on a large enough scale, man's health will be adversely affected.

Opponents of this viewpoint contend that soil fertility influences only the size of the crop and that the nutritional quality of a plant is determined primarily by genetic factors, notably the variety of seed that the farmer selects for his crop. If urban man is to exercise any control over the factors that influence his health, it is important that he gain some degree of familiarity with these problems. He need not get involved in technicalities, but he must acquire a general knowledge of soil needs and the relationship between soil fertility and the nutritional quality of crops.

Despite the sentiment and fervor ordinarily evoked by the words "land" and "soil," many people think of soil either as "dirt," a term that is often used synonymously with "filth," or as an inorganic resource, such as copper and iron. These misconceptions have not been completely eliminated by science. The rudiments of a science of soil were established in 1840, when Justus von Liebig published his monumental studies of soil and plant chemistry. Liebig had a profound grasp of his subject. He swept away many alchemistic notions about plant growth and replaced the more doubtful agricultural precepts of his day with new ones based on careful reasoning and scientific research. But Liebig also gave support to a misconception about soil that has yet to be completely removed from the public mind. He fostered the belief that soils are "lifeless storage bins filled with pulverized rocks, which held water and nutrients and which farmers stirred in tillage."

Agronomists generally agree that Liebig's conception of soil is incorrect. Although some soil scientists still hope to manipulate the soil as though it were little more than a reservoir of inorganic nutrients, few, if any, accept Liebig's approach. The soil is a palpitating sheet of life, varying in composition not only from one part of a country to another but from acre to acre. Man can analyze the soil but he cannot manufacture it. The first difficulty he encounters is its highly dynamic character and its remarkable complexity. The soil is a highly differentiated world of living and inanimate things, of vegetable and animal matter in various stages of decomposition, and of rock particles, minerals, water, and air. Soil is always in the process of formation. It gives up its nutrients to the wind, rain, and plants, and is replenished by the breakdown of rocks, the putrefaction of dead animals and plants, and the never-ending activities of microscopic life. The soil is the dramatic arena where life and death complement each other, where decay nourishes regeneration.

The surface soil, where most of the dead matter in soil is concentrated, is not the end product of decay; it is an active stage in the decomposition of organic matter. The decaying process, continually renewed by the addition of dead organisms, is as necessary for the continued existence of the soil as it is for the formation of soil. Humus, the black or brown organic portion of the soil, is a protoplasmic, jellylike substance made up of cells, leaves, and tissues that have lost their original structure. If humus were not renewed by the remains of dead organisms, the soil as we know it would disappear. The land surface of the earth would eventually be occupied by mineral particles and rocks, and the land would be inhospitable to advanced forms of plant and animal life.

Soil is made up of not only dead matter but living organisms. The most important of these organisms are either invisible or barely visible to the naked eye. Fungi, which initiate decomposition, and bacteria, which supply plants with usable nitrogen, are as much a part of the soil as humus and rock particles. These soil microbes supply most of the nitrogen required for plant growth. Their work is supplemented by the activities of countless insects and earthworms, which burrow elaborate galleries through the topsoil. Without the air that these galleries provide, plant nutrition would be inhibited and bacteria would be confined to the top few inches of the soil. Earthworms continually circulate soil nutrients. During a single year they may turn up as much as twenty tons of soil to the acre, burrowing to a depth of as much as six feet below the surface. As organic nutrients pass through their bodies, they leave behind casts that give the soil increased granularity and improve its ability to support plant life.

Soil would be washed or blown away if it were not held together internally. Its connective tissue, indeed its skeleton, is made up of the root systems of the plant life it supports. Roots reach out in all directions, intertwining with one another to form a living grillage beneath the surface of the land. By interlocking and binding soil granules in a network of root branches, they increase the soil's ability to withstand the impact of rain and wind. Above the surface, the forest's canopy of branches and leaves breaks rainfall into a fine spray. The erosive run-off so often encountered in open, sloping land is changed into a gentle flow that makes it possible for much of the water to be absorbed by the subsoil. The soil is spared and the water table is kept high. Finally, when plants die, their remains not only increase the fertility of the soil but also improve its structure. Lignin in roots, stalks, and trunks keeps the soil porous and friable—structural characteristics that favor the penetration of water and air.

In addition to microorganisms, soil fauna, and plants, the fourth major factor in the maintenance and formation of soils is the activity of large terrestrial animals on the surface. Under natural conditions, the land teems with wildlife, which leaves behind organic wastes rich in plant nutrients. Nature, as Sir Albert Howard has emphasized, is a mixed farmer: "Plants are always found with animals; many species of plants and animals live together." Nature seldom cultivates a single crop to the exclusion of all others. Variety and combination, of both plants and animals, constitute the basis for natural equilibrium. Herbivorous animals supply the topsoil with fecal matter; carnivores, in turn, regulate the number of plant eaters and thereby prevent excessive grazing. Normally, predators and their prey live in equilibrium. Rarely does it happen in the natural course of events that either group attains such numbers as to become pests and injure the soil.

Every plot of land should be viewed as a small, highly individuated cosmos. Merely identifying the organisms that promote the welfare of the soil does not adequately describe the dependence of each group on all the others. The performance of bacteria, it has been noted, depends in part on the capillary-like channels opened up by the passage of insects and earthworms through the soil. Insects and earthworms, in turn, depend for nutrients on the organic wastes of plants and animals. If the soil is structurally and nutritionally conducive to a balanced, thriving soil fauna, bacteria tend to penetrate further; topsoil becomes deeper and richer; plant growth becomes healthier and more luxuriant. When plants are abundant, wildlife is better nourished and more plentiful. If any external element disrupts this cosmos, the soil deteriorates and the living things that occupy the surface are adversely affected.

As long as man is a food gatherer or a hunter, he exercises a minor influence on the soil. He acquires what he needs where he finds it, and generally he has little effect upon the natural world. When he begins to cultivate the land, however, he imposes a new and often largely synthetic environment on his natural one. The soil cosmos is altered drastically. On forest lands, a large part of the indigenous tree cover is removed and the soil is exposed to the direct assaults of rain and wind. With the restriction of animal life, the return of manure to the land becomes fortuitous. Whether the soil is properly fertilized or not depends upon man's foresight, which is usually limited to serving his short-term economic interests. Lastly, the cultivation of a single plant species on a given tract of land tends to become the prevalent practice, and the checks and balances afforded by a diversity of vegetation are removed. The success of agriculture depends upon the extent to which man preserves the soil cosmos he inherits from nature. If the elements are merely rearranged and adequate compensation is made for necessary changes, the cultivation of food can continue indefinitely without harm to the soil; in fact, virgin soil can be improved immeasurably. But if the soil cosmos is undermined, soil will begin to disappear and the land will be forced to function with, as it were, its vital organs exposed and half its viscera removed.

The results can be disastrous. History supplies us with numerous accounts of civilizations that disappeared solely because of poor agricultural practices. Throughout the Mediterranean world, vast man-made deserts have supplanted rich, fertile lands that once nourished luxuriant crops and supported large populations. In North Africa, for example, a terrible price has been paid for the ancient plantation economy, in which land was cultivated for a few cash crops. The Phoenician merchants who established Carthage found a semi-arid but highly fertile soil on the southern shores of the Mediterranean Sea. Almost at the outset, farming assumed a highly commercialized form. A large acreage was irrigated and cultivated by slaves, and crops were planted and harvested primarily for the money they would bring in. "The intensive plantation cultivation which the Carthaginian plantation-owner undertook, and which was subsequently imitated by the Roman conquerors of the land, had the long-term effect of letting in the desert," Edward Hyams writes. "Conceivably, the original forest—and grass—soil communities might have acted as a barrier to the advancing sand, might have even pushed slowly southward, carrying a more humid climate with them as trees invaded the grass, and colonized the Sahara. But cultivation which took no account of soil as such, and was concerned with getting the largest possible crops out of the soil, had the opposite effect. The Sahara began its northward march; it has been on the move ever since; it has already invaded Europe, by way of Spain, an old African trick."

It is not difficult to see that the agricultural practices that reduced fertile areas of the Mediterranean world to a desert are being repeated today, especially in many areas of the United States. Both the forms and the effects are often the same. Modern agriculture tends to model itself on industry. Tens of thousands of acres are planted and harvested on a factory schedule, in some cases to meet the daily production requirements of a nearby food-processing plant. Every method that will "hurry along" cultivation and reduce its cost is eagerly seized upon. Food cultivation is rigorously standardized, even "time-studied." The division of labor in agriculture is developed to a point where the term "farmer" becomes a most general expression, applicable to pilots who spray insecticides from the air, truck and tractor drivers who merely operate vehicles, mechanics who repair farm implements, foremen who manage workers, and underprivileged migratory laborers, working at piece rates, who view the needs of the land with complete indifference. Husbandry is almost entirely subordinated to mass production. The modern land factory, like the metropolis that it feeds, tries to base the management of living things on a pernicious average. It employs primarily those methods that promote mass manipulation at the lowest cost.

Practices of this sort are as harmful to soil as they are to men. Modern agriculture often demands the largest possible farm machinery to handle its huge crops; heavy tractors move over the same area of land repeatedly—planting, spreading fertilizer, and harvesting crops. Although the use of machines in the performance of arduous tasks is certainly desirable from a human point of view, every mechanical advance should be properly scaled, both in size and form, to the situation at hand. The land is not the concrete floor of a factory; it is a living thing, and it can be mauled and bruised. Injury to the soil, often of a serious nature, inevitably follows the exposure of fields to the weight of extraordinarily heavy machines. The soil becomes compacted, and as a result, proper drainage and the growth of roots are inhibited. Data from Texas indicate that crop yields of compacted soils there have fallen off from 40 to 50 per cent, and commercial fertilizers have not been able to increase the yields to any great extent. "After 100 years of farm-implement development," observes Howard W. Lull, of the

U. S. Forestry Service, "more than half of Germany's cultivated soils are in poor condition—due largely to compaction by tractors. In Great Britain, the rapid increase in the weight of tractors in recent years has led to predictions of serious effects on the soil."

The deterioration of soil is carried further when large areas of land are used to cultivate a single crop. The land factory separates not only animal from plant, but plant from plant. Precisely where plant and animal wastes are most needed to help the soil withstand the weight of heavy machinery, a strong emphasis is placed on one-crop agriculture and industrial methods. The structure of the soil breaks down and the layer of humus begins to disappear. In many areas of the United States, the land has been turned into a nearly lifeless, inorganic medium that must be nursed along like an invalid at the threshold of death.

The term "inorganic medium" can be taken literally. Modern agriculture may be distinguished from earlier forms of cultivation by its reliance on chemistry for soil nutrients and the control of insect infestations. With the removal of many natural checks and balances, we are compelled to use many synthetic materials to grow and protect our foods. These chemical agents enable us to produce large crops on indifferent and even poor soils. The ultimate is reached with hydroponics, which uses no soil at all. An open box is filled with pebbles and a solution of inorganic nutrients. Then seeds or roots are placed directly in the medium, or sometimes seeds are supported in the solution by a wire screen until they germinate and sink their roots into the pebbles. With adequate light, proper temperature, and the appropriate renewal of inorganic nutrients, the plants mature rapidly and become an edible crop.

In an age of demonstrable scientific achievement, it

is hardly necessary to emphasize the agricultural importance of chemistry. Chemical analysis has advanced our knowledge of the soil cosmos and plant nutrition enormously, and there is no a priori reason why man-made chemical agents cannot be used to considerable advantage in increasing the fertility of the soil. Soil is fertilized to increase the quantity and quality of food crops. Wherever man acquires the knowledge and the chemical agents to achieve these ends, he enjoys a decisive advantage over less-developed agricultural communities. Natural processes can be rendered more efficient and some of the life lines that determine the abundance and quality of plants can be shortened, both to the advantage of man and the organisms on whose well-being he depends. If rational standards were applied to agriculture, it would be possible for farmers to systematically meet various needs of the land that would probably have remained unsatisfied if the solution of soil problems had been left to natural processes alone.

But there is a danger that the techniques of modern chemistry will be abused. This danger is especially pronounced in an age of scientific achievement, in which a limited amount of knowledge tends to create the illusion that our command of the agricultural situation is complete and our standards of agricultural success are rational. Modern society places a strong emphasis on the merits of mass production. We tend to confuse quantity with quality. The thoughtless use of chemical agents in the production of food may well make it possible to grow crops of great abundance but of low quality on soil that is basically in poor condition. "High yields are not . . . synonymous with a high content of nutrient elements," observes A. G. Norman, of the University of Michigan. "Crops from well fertilized plots may have a lower content of some essential elements than those from poorly yielding plots, the addition of a fertilizer may cause a reduction in content of some of the other nutrient elements, or, if the supply of the major elements is such that the content of each in the plant falls in the poverty adjustment zone [where a partial deficiency of nutrients exists], moderate addition of one of them may have rather little effect on content."

Without making a fetish of nature, a number of responsible agronomists and conservationists doubt strongly whether a basically poor soil is capable of meeting all the nutritional requirements of plants, animals, and man with the support of a few chemical fertilizers. "In the long run life cannot be supported, so far as our present knowledge goes, by artificial processes," observes Fairfield Osborn, a noted American conservationist. "The deterioration of the life-giving elements of the earth, that is proceeding at a constantly accelerating velocity, may be checked but cannot be cured by man-applied chemistry." Osborn sees two basic reasons why "artificial processes, unless they are recognized as complements to natural processes, will fail to provide the solution" to current soil and health problems. "The first is concerned with the actual nature of productive soils," by which is meant the complexity of the soil cosmos. "The second reason is a practical one and hinges upon the difficulty, if not impossibility, of instructing great numbers of people who work on the land regarding the extremely complicated techniques that need to be applied to produce even a reasonable degree of fertility by artificial methods."

Whatever one may think of Osborn's conclusions, the issue is obviously of great importance in any discussion of environmental health, and it raises the additional question of one's approach to our synthetic environment. Knowledge is never absolute. What we "know" about anything, be it soil or nutrition, generally consists of the facts that are selected for our purpose. If our objectives are comprehensive, so too will be the data they command. If they are limited, the data adduced in their support may entail a suppression, conscious or unconscious, of facts that support broader objectives. The physician who is burdened with a schematic conception of disease is inclined to ignore subtle functions of the body whose impairment contributes to the incidence of chronic and degenerative illnesses. Similarly, the agriculturist who is guided primarily by such quantitative criteria as the size of the crops is inclined to ignore ecological processes whose impairment may lower the nutritional quality of food. The evidence that both adduce in support of their views, such as man's greater longevity and larger crops, does not prove that man's longer life span is the result of better health or that the abundant crop is greater in food value.

The tendency to place the soil on a limited ration of chemical fertilizers becomes stronger with each passing year. Nearly a decade ago, George L. McNew, of the Boyce Thompson Institute for Plant Research, observed that the quantity of inorganic fertilizers used in agriculture had increased over 200 per cent between the prewar years and 1948. "Less barnyard manure is being added to the soil each year. Not enough green manure from cover crops is being plowed under to maintain the organic matter content in soils on most of our farms." The implications of this change in agricultural methods call for sober consideration. We must closely examine the way in which current fertilization practices are likely to affect the nutritional quality of food, especially in circumstances where economic incentives are likely to make misuses of chemicals the rule rather than the exception.

SOIL FERTILITY AND NUTRITION

BEFORE WE CAN UNDERSTAND the role that soil fertility plays in environmental health, an important question must be answered. Do we have a complete knowledge of the nutritive constituents of common foods and do we fully understand the function that all the known nutrients have in the human body? Many researchers in the field of nutrition and in related sciences agree that the answer is no. "There is no known laboratory method or group of methods by which all the nutritive constituents in a food can be measured and evaluated in terms of the nutrition of man or animals," observes Kenneth C. Beeson, formerly director of the Department of Agriculture's Plant, Soil, and Nutrition Laboratory. ". . . All of the constituents contributing to nutritive quality have probably not been recognized and there are no adequate methods for quantitative measure in many constituents that we do recognize."

The same problem is stated very clearly by Bruce Bliven in a popular discussion of hydroponics. "We do not know whether we have yet enumerated the entire list of chemicals and other substances necessary for the maintenance of health and vigor. The 'trace minerals' that occur in minute quantities in our food, including cobalt, copper, phosphorus, manganese, iodine, and others, are known to be of enormous importance to health, though we are not yet sure just how many of them are required, or in what quantities. We do not even know how many vitamins there are, or which are essential. Theoretically, it should be possible to produce fruits and vegetables from soil that is lacking in some of the substances necessary for the health of animals and man; these fruits and vegetables would look all right, and yet prove to be harmful if they were a principal part of the diet."

The possibility of producing plants that "look all right" but vary widely in nutritional values is more than theoretical; such cultivation is eminently practical and very common. Identical varieties of vegetables, fruit, and grain may differ appreciably in mineral, protein, and vitamin content. These variations are caused by many factors, a number of which are not within man's control. For example, the vitamin-C content of fruit and leafy vegetables seems to depend primarily upon the amount of sunshine to which the plants are exposed. Variations in temperature influence the production of thiamine and carotene in different plant species. The longer the growing season, the greater will be the amount of vitamin C in beans, spinach, and lettuce. Aside from these climatic and seasonal factors, however, a decisive role in plant nutrition is played by soil fertility. Despite sharp differences of opinion that have developed around the issue of soil and nutrition, a large amount of evidence supports the conclusion that the nutritional quality of plants is influenced profoundly by the fertility of the soil.

This influence may be beneficial or undesirable, depending upon the type and quantity of fertilizer used in any given agricultural situation. In general, nitrogen fertilizer tends to increase the proportion of crude protein in grain. This relationship has been established in several experiments. During the late 1940's, research by R. L. Lovern and M. F. Miller at the University of Missouri showed that the percentage of crude protein in one variety of wheat could be raised from a minimum of 8.9 to a maximum of 17 by successive applications of soluble nitrogen to the soil. Three years of experimental work by A. S. Hunter and his co-workers on 133 farms in the Columbia Basin counties of Oregon indicated that applications of nitrogen fertilizer usually increase the amount of protein in pastry-type wheats. Results of a similar nature have also been achieved with corn. H. E. Sauberlich and his colleagues at the Alabama Agricultural Experiment Station cultivated two grades of corn—a "low protein" grain (6.8 to 9.1 per cent) and a "high protein" grain (9.5 to 13.6 per cent). The "high protein" corn was produced by increasing the application of nitrogen fertilizer to the soil.

When agronomists turn their attention from the protein to the mineral constituents of plants, they find that soil fertility exercises a more subtle influence on nutritive quality. The addition of calcium, phosphorus, potassium, and other nutrients to depleted soils often increases the mineral content of plants; but the experiments do not yield consistent results. In many cases an increase does not take place. In fact, if the soil is not deficient in common minerals, attempts to increase yields by adding high concentrations of commercial fertilizers to the soil may actually reduce the nutritive quality of plants. The soil may become "over-fertilized," and the quantity of important nutrients in the crop will diminish.

How are these contradictory results to be explained? A partial answer is provided by the findings of soil chemistry and plant physiology. Many factors may inhibit a plant's uptake and utilization of a nutrient. Research workers have discovered that an excessive quantity of one nutrient in the soil may prevent the absorption and utilization of another. "Too much nitrogen, for example, in proportion to the phosphorus available to plants, may encourage undesirable physiological conditions. Also too much calcium may interfere with phosphorus and boron nutrition or may encourage chlorosis [lack of chlorophyll] due to a reduction in the availability of the soil iron, zinc, or manganese." Several key nutrients have been paired together on the basis of such interactions, notably calcium and magnesium, iron and manganese, and cobalt and manganese. Moreover, it would be incorrect to assume that a simple one-to-one relationship exists between available soil nitrogen and the protein content of plants. Proteins differ markedly in nutritional value. By applying excessive quantities of commercial nitrogen fertilizer to the soil, a farmer may well produce a lush crop that contains less high-quality and more low-quality proteins than crops cultivated on properly fertilized soils. An objective review of the evidence at hand not only justifies the conclusion that soil fertility influences the nutritive quality of food; it also leads us to believe that this influence is more complex and more subtle than was formerly suspected. A balanced array of nutrients, modified where necessary to satisfy the needs of a specific soil, is indispensable to the cultivation of highly nutritious crops.

At a time when many farmers are trying to cultivate large crops by supplying the soil with a few highly concentrated inorganic fertilizers, it would be appropriate to emphasize the important role that organic matter plays in plant nutrition as well as in the reconstruction of soil. Organic matter is extremely complex and highly varied in nutritional content. Manure, for example, will not only supply soil with adequate quantities of nitrogen released by microbes in close accord with the plant's needs; it will also add most of the nutrients that plants require for growth and well-being. No one seriously claims that manure alone meets all the needs of a crop, but its array of nutrients is probably unequaled by the commercial fertilizer preparations that are normally used today.

The use of organic fertilizers has often made the difference between successful food cultivation and outright crop failures. Until well into the 1920's, many American agronomists were convinced that soil merely required heavy dosages of nitrogen, phosphorus, and potassium—the well-known NPK formula—to produce flourishing crops. These elements, it was supposed, were all that organic fertilizers contributed to plant nutrition. When inexpensive commercially prepared fertilizers became available, nitrogen, phosphorus, and potassium compounds replaced manures, bone meal, and plant residues. Serious crop failures often followed the changeover. In Florida, for example, nutritional deficiencies appeared in citrus and tung trees; they were corrected by a return to the use of organic matter. Intensive research disclosed that bone meal supplied citrus trees with sorely needed magnesium in quantities that were not provided by the inorganic compounds in use at the time. Fortunately, the deficiency appeared in an acute form; it was easily discovered and later corrected by new chemical agents. But success in correcting acute nutritional deficiencies is likely to lower our guard against insidious deficiencies that may not manifest themselves as clearcut plant disorders. Many plants may require nutrients in amounts that are not supplied by commonly used inorganic preparations.

The majority of commercial fertilizers in use today are relatively simple chemical preparations. The farmer deliberately replaces complex, bulky, slow-acting organic materials with a few soluble, purified, inexpensive, and easily handled salts. The regulation of soil fertility now falls for the most part to man. "The agronomist and the farmer are ordinarily preoccupied with yield," Norman writes. "They are rarely concerned with mineral composition. The varieties selected, the cultural practices followed, the fertilizers applied, all are decided on the basis of yield expectation." The manipulation of soil fertility in accordance with this criterion may produce very curious results. For example, in studies conducted at the Missouri Agricultural Experiment Station, it was found that by changing the ratio of calcium to potassium, it was possible to increase the vegetative bulk of soybeans by one fourth. "Such increased tonnage would warrant agronomic applause," observes William A. Albrecht, of the University of Missouri. "But this increase in vegetative mass represented a reduction in the concentration of protein by one fourth, a reduction in the concentration of phosphorus by one half and a reduction in the concentration of calcium by two thirds over that in the smaller tonnage yield" produced by a different ratio of calcium to potassium.

Although heavy applications of NPK fertilizer to the soil often produce lush, abundant forage, the crop may be very deficient in key nutrients. Beeson presents a summary of an interesting experiment by H. A. Keener and E. J. Thacker at the New Hampshire Agricultural Experiment Station that clearly illustrates this point. "Excellent yields of brome-ladino or timothy hay produced in New Hampshire with high level applications of fertilizer have failed to provide an adequate forage for calves. Deficiency symptoms observed in calves are poor growth, rough coats, anemia, sagging of the spinal column behind the shoulders, an ataxia [lack of co-ordination] of the hind legs (timothy-fed calves only), loss of tips of ears, and broken bones." Supplements of copper and iron did not remove any of these symptoms. When similar hay was fed to rabbits, the same deficiency symptoms appeared.

A chemical analysis of samples from the crop would not have disclosed the complete extent of the deficiency. At first Keener and Thacker suspected that the "timothy hay was deficient in iodine and one or more organic factors," but later studies by Thacker showed that the "deficiency in the hay was related to its mineral composition." Similar experiments have led many agronomists to conclude that the nutritional value of a crop must be judged primarily by the response of the organism that consumes it, not merely by chemical analyses of the soil and the plant.

If the adequacy of our agricultural methods is judged by the health of our livestock, then American agriculture must be regarded as a failure. The health of our domestic animals has been deteriorating noticeably for years. Veterinary medicine has been able to reduce the incidence of infectious diseases in livestock and poultry primarily because of new antibiotic preparations, but the resistance of the animals is very low. The number of cattle with cancers of the lymph and blood-forming organs that are being condemned at federally inspected packing plants has increased from 9.2 per 100,000 in 1950 to 18.2 in 1959, nearly 100 per cent in nine years; during the same period the number of swine condemned for similar cancers rose 97 per cent. Sterility in animals is arousing deep concern. "The most important problem in the beef industry is poor reproductive performance, as evidenced by low percentage calf crops," note a group of investigators at the Beltsville Experiment Station in Maryland.* The ubiquitous environmental changes of our time seem to have affected animal life as profoundly as they have affected man.

Every problem, to be sure, should be placed in its proper setting. The use of highly concentrated chemical

---

* The experimental work reported by these investigators shows that diet is a prime factor in the reproductive performance of animals. By increasing, decreasing, or changing the composition of the ration, the Beltsville researchers found that beef cows respond with remarkable variations in fertility, sexual activity, and the ability to deliver offspring. A moderate but balanced ration of carbohydrates and proteins yielded the highest reproductive rates.

fertilizers and mass-production techniques increases agricultural output at relatively small cost and with little effort. If the purpose of growing food is to prevent famine and acute nutritional disorders, these methods produce immediate results. They satisfy the dire need for food, and they remove the more obvious diseases produced by an inadequate diet. But if we enlarge our view of modern agriculture to include such problems as the quality of food and the health of plants, livestock, and human beings, the success that is ordinarily claimed for current agricultural techniques requires qualification. Man does not practice agriculture in a vacuum. His activities as a cultivator of food are influenced more by his forms of social organization than by his solicitude for the needs of the soil. The majority of American farmers, large and small, cultivate food as a business enterprise. They try to produce large crops at a minimum cost. As it may well be difficult to increase the output of the soil without lowering the quality of crops, the farmer who places quality above quantity can scarcely hope to survive the competitive demands of American agriculture. Accordingly, we can expect any technique that promotes large crops to be carried to the point of abuse. Economic competition leaves the farmer little choice but to replace low standards of food cultivation with even lower ones.

It is highly probable that exploitation of the soil has already produced a deterioration in the nutritive quality of crops in many parts of the United States. William A. Albrecht, one of America's most perceptive and creative agronomists, suggests that more carbohydrates and fewer high-quality proteins tend to appear in our food staples with the passage of time. The extent of this shift in nutritive quality is difficult to determine. Commercial foods are generally graded according to appearance, and very little attention is given to nutritive quality. The information that is available, however, is not encouraging. Albrecht has pointed out that between 1940 and 1949 the concentration of protein in Kansas-grown corn declined from 9.5 to 8.5 per cent, although the decade was marked by substantial increases in corn yields. "It is interesting to note the reduction in the protein content of corn as reported in successive editions of a standard handbook of feeds and feeding. In the Eleventh Edition, published 40 years ago, the only figure quoted for crude protein of dent corn was 10.3 per cent. In the Twenty-First edition, 1950, five grades of corn were cited, for which the protein figures ranged from 8.8 to 7.9, with a mean of nearly 8.4 per cent. During the interval of 40 years between the two editions, crude protein in corn dropped from 10.3 to 8.4, a reduction of 22 per cent."

There also seems to be evidence of an over-all decline in the protein content of Kansas-grown wheat. "A survey of the percentage protein of Kansas wheat grain made in 1940 showed a range of 10 to almost 19 per cent," Albrecht notes. "In a similar survey ten years later, in 1949, protein concentration was found to range from 9 to less than 15 per cent."

We can ill afford such losses. At a time when many individuals are consuming substantially more food than they require for the work they do, an increase in carbohydrates at the expense of proteins is obviously undesirable, particularly for middle-aged people. Great importance should be attached to the quality of the food we consume. We are continually being reminded that there is a close connection between obesity and chronic diseases. An overweight individual has a greater chance of acquiring cancer, diabetes, and cardiovascular disorders than one who maintains his proper weight. Any shift in the

quality of foods that results in an increase of carbohydrates can be expected to contribute to the erosion of
public health.

Viewing nutritional problems in a broader perspective, it is difficult to believe that human fitness can be
maintained while the soil is gradually deteriorating. Albrecht observes: "Man has become aware of increased
needs for health preservation, interpreted as a technical
need for more hospitals, drugs, and doctors, when it may
simply be a matter of failing to recognize the basic truth
in the old adage which reminded us that 'to be well fed
is to be healthy.' Unfortunately, we have not seen the
changes man has wrought in his soil community in terms
of food quality for health, as economics and technologies
have emphasized its quantity. Man is exploiting the earth
that feeds him much as a parasite multiplies until it kills
its host. Slowly the reserves in the soil for the support of
man's nutrition are being exhausted. All too few of us
have yet seen the soil community as the foundation in
terms of nutrition of the entire biotic pyramid of which,
man, at the top, occupies the most hazardous place."

ENVIRONMENT AND ECOLOGICAL PATTERNS

THERE IS A CLOSE RELATIONSHIP between modern concepts of progress and man's attempt to control the forces
of nature. From the time of the Renaissance, man has
tended to evaluate nearly all the advances of society and
science in terms of the amount of power over the natural
world which they gave him. The word "power," however,
has many shades of meaning. To the men of the Renaissance and the Enlightenment, it would have seemed pre-

posterous that power over nature meant more than living in harmony with the natural world. Like the animals around him, man was a product of natural forces and depended upon nature for his survival and well-being. What made him unique in the animal kingdom was his ability to reason. This faculty gave him the power to remove fortuity from his relationship to nature, to bring a certain degree of guidance to natural processes. He could try to mitigate the harshness of the natural world and make the interplay of natural forces relatively benign. Power over nature was regarded as the ability of man to enter into *conscious* symbiosis with the biotic world.

With the Industrial Revolution, the concept of power over nature underwent a radical change. The word "nature" was replaced by the phrase "natural resources." The new captains of industry regarded land, forests, and wildlife as materials for wanton exploitation. The progress of man was identified with the pillage of nature. The needs of commerce and industry produced a new ideology: There are no dictates of nature that are beyond human transgression. Technology, it was claimed, is capable of giving man complete mastery over the natural world. If these notions seem naïve today, it is because the needless, often senseless, conflict between man and nature is yielding unexpected consequences. We are now learning that the more man works against nature, the more deeply entangled he becomes in the very forces he seeks to master.

The problems created by our conflict with nature are dramatically exemplified by our chemical war against the insect world. During the past two decades, a large number of insecticides have been developed for general use on farms and in the home. The best-known and most widely used preparations are the chlorinated hydrocarbons, such as DDT, methoxychlor, dieldrin, and chlordane. The chlorinated hydrocarbons are sprayed over vast acres of forest land, range land, crop land, and even semi-urban land on which there are heavy infestations of insects. It is doubtful whether any part of the United States with some kind of vegetation useful to man has not been treated at least once in the past ten years. Most of our fields and orchards are sprayed recurrently during the growing season. Aside from the hazards that insecticides create for public health, many conservationists claim that extensive use of the new insecticides is impairing the ability of wildlife and beneficial insects to exercise control over pests. They point out that the insecticides are taking a heavy toll of life among fish, birds, small mammals, and useful insects. There is a great deal of evidence that the new chemicals are self-defeating. Not only have they failed to eradicate most of the pests against which they are employed; in some cases, new pests and greater infestations have been created as a result of the damage inflicted on predators of species formerly under control.

To understand this problem clearly, it is necessary to examine the conditions that promote infestations of pests. A species becomes a pest when it invades a new area that is not inhabited by its natural enemies or when environmental changes occur that provide more favorable conditions for its growth. Under natural conditions, infestations are episodic and rare. An increase in the pest species creates propitious conditions for those predators that live on the pest. The proliferation of the pest encourages the proliferation of its predators and attracts additional enemies from nearby regions. Whichever way the problem is solved, the remarkable diversity and adaptability of life under natural conditions seldom permit the pest to get completely out of hand.

Insect infestations become persistent and serious, however, when natural variety is diminished by man.

Agriculture, especially when limited to one crop, tends to simplify a natural region. "The first person to harvest and store natural cereal grain for later sowing started the simplification of agriculture," observes Robert L. Rudd, of the University of California. "Until the mechanization and later chemicalization of agriculture, there was little substantial departure from the methods of the first agriculturalists. Acreages were small, landscapes diverse." The simplification of ecological systems "was relatively slight and was in any event local. Hedgerows, trees, weed patches, seasonal cropping and multipurpose farming combined to form a diversified base for a diversified fauna. Mechanized and chemicalized crop production has resulted in large expanses of single crop species—the destruction of diversity in the landscape."

Simplification of the landscape, followed by a diminution in the variety of fauna, creates highly favorable conditions for an infestation. A potential pest is left with a large food supply and a small number of predators. The job of eradicating the pest, like that of fertilizing the soil, falls primarily to man, and thus far the methods employed and the results achieved have been very unsatisfactory. Man can usually eradicate a pest—but only for a while. In the process, he often eradicates nearly every other form of life in the area aside from the crop. When the pest returns, as it often does, the ecological system may have been so simplified by the pesticidal treatment that the new conditions are more favorable for infestation than the old. "Initial chemical control, therefore, creates the later need for more chemicals," Rudd adds. "Once begun, there is no stopping if the crop is not to be lost."

Many responsible conservationists regard the nonselective spraying of open land and forests as an ecological "boomerang." In a number of cases, the damage inflicted on beneficial insects outweighs the damage inflicted on the pest. Pesticidal treatments have started infestations that would have been very mild, if not averted entirely, had the treatment not been used. In one region, for example, the treatment of a stand of timber with a five-pound-per-acre dosage of DDT in early summer resulted in a general infestation of at least fourteen species of aphids. The aphids, clinging to the undersurface of the leaves, survived the spray, but their predators were decimated and failed to re-establish themselves rapidly enough to check the infestation. In still other cases, controlled insects have been transformed into serious pests by the destruction of their predators through spraying programs aimed at an entirely different species of pest. For example, until fairly recently the red-banded leaf roller caused very little damage in apple orchards. Although widely distributed, the insect was strictly controlled by parasites and predators. "Rare indeed was the orchardist who knowingly had to contend with it," writes Howard Baker, of the Bureau of Entomology. "Now it is a problem pest throughout the Midwest and East, where in 1947 and 1948 particularly it caused severe damage in many orchards." The insect became a pest after its parasites had been destroyed by DDT. To control the leaf roller, orchardists are now compelled to supplement DDT treatments with TDE and parathion. "Never before . . . have so many pests with such a wide range of habits and characteristics increased to injurious levels following application of any one material as has occurred following the use of DDT in apple spray programs."

Non-selective spraying programs are taking a heavy toll of life among birds and rodents—animals that play a major role in limiting infestations of harmful insects. Although rodents are generally regarded as little more than pests themselves, forest rodents are voracious consumers of insects. On an average, insects constitute 20 per cent of the diet of forest mice, chipmunks, and flying squirrels. The importance of birds in insect control scarcely requires emphasis. Suffice it to say that naturalists who have made careful counts of insects in the stomachs of birds have found, for example, 5,000 ants in a flicker, 500 mosquitoes in a night hawk, and 250 tent caterpillers in a yellow-billed cuckoo. A brown thrasher will eat more than 6,000 insects in a single day; a swallow, about 1,000 leaf hoppers. Spraying commonly destroys an appreciable number of these creatures, even when the program is fairly limited in scope. To cite a case in point: In 1956 the Cranbrook Institute of Science, in Michigan, undertook a limited survey of the decline in bird life produced by DDT spraying programs to control the Dutch elm disease. Residents of the immediate area were asked to turn in or report to the Institute any birds suspected of having been poisoned by DDT. "During April, May and June of that year, but mostly in May, more than 200 dead and dying birds were turned in to the Institute. . . . By 1959 the number of specimens received had mounted to about 400, with an estimated 600 calls or reports regarding birds not turned in." A survey of the bird life on the Cranbrook campus showed that the breeding population declined from 250 pairs to 25 or less. Most of the dead and dying birds were robins that were probably poisoned by eating worms impregnated with DDT.

A more extensive survey was made during the widely publicized fire-ant campaign that the Department of Agriculture initiated in November 1957. The data, compiled by the National Audubon Society, deal with many animals, including more than a hundred head of cattle killed in an area near Climax, Georgia. We shall confine ourselves, however, to losses among birds. "The drastic effect of applying insecticide during the bird-nesting season was dramatically shown in Texas. In a 60-acre clover field bird numbers declined alarmingly: 38 of 41 nests with eggs were abandoned or destroyed. Lay's Texas report summarizes the devastating results tersely as follows: 'Bird populations along ranch roads in the treated areas were reduced 92-97 per cent in two weeks. Bird populations within acre plots studied were reduced 85 per cent in two weeks. Nesting success of birds in the area was reduced 89 per cent (compared with a non-treated area).' Lay adds, 'Large scale abandonment of nests with eggs could be explained only by the mortality of the adults. The missing birds did not appear in adjacent areas.' "

To aggravate the damage, insecticides are carried by surface and ground water into streams and lakes, where they kill large numbers of aquatic animals. For example, one pound of dieldrin per acre, applied to a large tract of land in St. Lucie County, Florida, destroyed twenty to thirty tons of fish. During 1958, a DDT campaign against the spruce budworm in northern Maine killed thousands of trout and other game fish; as long as three months after spraying, trout were found whose bodies contained DDT concentrations of from 2.9 to 198 parts per million. The sprayers were not entirely unaware of what the consequences of the program would be. Two years earlier a campaign of much the same kind produced heavy losses of young salmon in the nearby Miramichi River system of New Brunswick, Canada. "As expected, an alarmingly reduced adult Atlantic salmon run was noted in 1960 when the 1956 hatch returned to spawn in the Miramichi River system."

The discovery of DDT led to a widespread belief that insect pests could be eradicated by relying exclusively on the use of chemical agents. This belief was severely shaken when it was found that a number of harmful species were producing strains that were resistant to

existing insecticides, and now many entomologists suspect that the appearance of such strains in nearly all
major species of pests is merely a matter of time. As
long as present methods of control are employed, new
insecticides will be required every few years just to hold
the line in man's chemical war against the insect world.
The appearance of resistant strains among man's most
formidable insect enemies has profound biological implications. In addition to all the harm man has inflicted
on the land and the biosphere, he is now becoming a
self-damaging selective force in the insect world. Insecticides do not make "the susceptible more resistant,"
A. W. A. Brown observes, "for they are dead. Rather, the
chemical had discovered the favored few that had a certain margin of resistance and selected them to survive and
breed. Normally they would be eliminated by parasites
and predators, to whom this kind of resistance means
nothing. But if the chemical treatment has removed the
biological control species, the more resistant individuals
of the pest species can survive to breed. . . . It is ironic
that the economic entomologist has thus been able to
speed up evolution to man's own disadvantage."

Brown's conclusion is an indictment of our methods
of dealing with the natural world. Biological evolution has
been governed not only by the survival of the fittest but
also by the ability of living things to assume an inex-
haustible variety of forms. The world of life has met every
change in climate and landscape with a more diversified
and interdependent biosphere. Each stage of organic evolution has been marked by a greater degree of specialization, complexity, and interrelatedness than the preceding
one. Almost every species that has been "selected" for
survival exhibits a higher order of specialization and depends for its continued existence upon a more complex
environment than its predecessors.

Modern man is undoing the work of organic evolution, replacing a complex environment with a simpler one. He is disassembling the biotic pyramid that has supported human life for countless millennia. Almost all the manifold relationships on which man's food plants and domestic animals depend for health are being replaced by more elementary relationships, and the biosphere is slowly being restored to a stage in which it will be able to support only a simpler form of life. It is not within the realm of fantasy to suggest that if the breakdown of the soil cosmos continues unabated, if plant and animal health continue to deteriorate, if insect infestations multiply, and if chemical controls become increasingly lethal, many of the preconditions for advanced life will be irreparably damaged and the earth will prove to be incapable of supporting a viable, healthy human species.

The simplification of man's environment has evoked deep concern among ecologists, particularly in connection with the insect problem. Only in the "conscious pitting of one living thing against another—biological control— can we directly control pests without the hazards accompanying repetitive chemical applications," Rudd writes. ". . . European entomologists now speak of managing the entire plant-insect community. It is called manipulation of the biocenose. The biocenetic environment is varied, complex and dynamic. Although numbers of individuals will constantly change, no one species will normally reach pest proportions. The special conditions which allow high populations of a single species in a complex ecosystem [a pattern of life] are rare events. Management of the biocenose or ecosystem should become our goal, challenging as it is."

Needless to say, the soil is no less an ecosystem than the complexes established by plants, insects, and animals.

When an agronomist emphasizes that organic matter is vital to the fertility of the soil, his emphasis derives from an appreciation of the manifold requirements of the soil cosmos and plant nutrition. Although organic matter is not a panacea for the ills of agriculture and human health, it provides good crops and it supplies plants with nutrients in a manner that has met the requirements of plant life over long ages of botanical evolution. The role played by chemical fertilizers in agriculture may be very important, especially in circumstances where animal and plant wastes are in short supply or where man's need for food is pressing. But the value of chemical fertilizers lies in their ability to complement the nutritional diversity of organic matter, not to supplant animal and plant wastes entirely.

An ecological point of view that emphasizes the use of organic materials and the practice of biocenetic control admittedly restricts man. It requires him to reconstruct the agricultural situation along more natural lines, to defer to the dictates of ecology rather than those of economics. To borrow the words of Charles Elton, this point of view is not intended "to promote any idea of complete *laissez faire* in the management of the ecosystems of the world. . . . The world's future has to be managed, but this management would not be just like a game of chess—more like steering a boat. We need to learn how to manipulate more wisely the tremendous potential forces of population growth in plants and animals, how to allow sufficient freedom for some of these forces to work amongst themselves, and how to grow environments . . . that will maintain a permanent balance in each community."

CHAPTER THREE

Urban Life and Health

THE CHANGING URBAN SCENE

MAN'S ENVIRONMENT attains a high degree
of simplification in the modern metropolis. At first this
may seem surprising: We normally associate metropolitan life with a diversity of individual types and with
variety and subtlety in human relations. But diversity
among men and complexity in human relations are
social and cultural phenomena. From a biological point
of view, the drab, severe metropolitan world of mortar,
steel, and machines constitutes a relatively simple environment, and the sharp division of labor developed by
the modern urban economy imposes extremely limited,
monotonous occupational activities on many of the individuals who make their livelihood in a large city.

These have not always been the characteristics of
urban life. The metropolitan milieu represents a sharp

departure from the forms and styles of life that prevailed in communities of the pre-industrial era. Early towns produced highly varied and colorful environments. Students of the medieval commune and the Renaissance city never fail to single out the humanizing artistic touch that the urban dweller gave to his home and to everyday articles. Craftsmen seldom permitted the function of an object to completely dominate its form. Decorativeness is to be found even in tools and weapons—objects which in our day are noteworthy for their purely functional design. This high sense of individual artistry was nourished by a vocational tradition that directed the workman to nearly every phase of the making of a product. The craftsman often prepared his raw material with his own hands, smelting his metals or tanning his leather. The great architects and engineers of the Renaissance not only designed a structure but also participated in its construction. The roundedness of the Renaissance man, which we look upon with so much envy today, was due in large part to a unity of mind and body, to a combination of thought and physical activity.

Early urban life was leisurely and relaxed. Craftsmen worked more or less in accordance with a pace established by physiological cycles, accelerating the tempo of their work during moments of energy and slowing down or halting entirely during periods of lethargy. The rate of physical activity was determined by the body's vitality rather than by external agencies, such as machines. Men did not try to "conserve" their energy and distribute it uniformly, as though it were an inorganic resource; human energy is seldom "conserved," in this simple, mechanical sense. Craftsman and artist worked by "fits and starts," giving themselves over to a task to the degree that their bodies were amenable to physical activity and artistic endeavor. Labor and art were seldom forced. The tempo of work varied, from hour to hour and day to day, with the changing vitality of the body.

The town developed in an agricultural matrix. Farms lay directly outside the city, not in a far-removed perimeter that the traveler could reach only after a long journey through suburbs and "exurbs." A short stroll carried the urban dweller from the market place, on which the principal cultural activities of the community were centered, into open fields and orchards. Farmer and city man intermingled freely. In many cases, the urban dweller combined the work of a craftsman with that of a food grower, often maintaining a small garden inside the city walls to supply some of his own food. "One must not look at the narrow streets between the houses without remembering the open green, or the neatly chequered gardens, that usually stretched behind," observes Lewis Mumford.

Food staples were grown nearby, on farms that produced a variety of crops. As soon as a crop was harvested, it found its way quickly to the market place and from there to the urban consumer. The city dweller was never completely urbanized, in the narrow sense, as he is today. Gardening within the city and easy access to the countryside helped to fuse all aspects of urban and country life.

Early city life, to be sure, was burdened with many problems that have largely been solved by modern science and technology. Diet was severely restricted, especially in medieval times, and fresh foods were available only during the growing season. Sanitation remained primitive for centuries, although Mumford points out that the existence of open spaces in the medieval town "shows that sanitary arrangements were not necessarily as offensive as they have been pictured, nor vile smells as uniformly ubiquitous." Agricultural techniques were crude and few advances were made in transportation until

railroads came into existence, but the early towns put
the tools and the knowledge at their disposal to the best
possible use. Life was usually serene. "One awoke in the
medieval town to the crowing of the cock, the chirping
of birds nesting under the eaves, or to the tolling of the
hours in the monastery on the outskirts, perhaps to the
chime of bells in the new belltower. Song rose easily on
the lips, from the plain chant of the monks to the re-
frains of the ballad singer in the market place, or that
of the apprentice and the house-maid at work. As late
as the seventeenth century, the ability to hold a part in
a domestic choral song was rated by Pepys as an indispensable quality in a new maid. There were work songs,
distinct for each craft, often composed to the rhythmic
tapping or hammering of the craftsman himself. Fitz-
Stephens reported in the twelfth century that the sound
of the water mill was a pleasant one amid the green
fields of London. At night there would be complete silence,
but for the stirring of animals and the calling of the
hours by the town watch. Deep sleep was possible in the
medieval towns, untainted by either human or mechanical
noises."

Modern science has eliminated nearly all the difficulties that earlier urban communities faced. Owing to
advanced means of transportation, the city dweller now
enjoys a highly varied diet, and the metropolis receives
abundant supplies of foods of all types the year round.
Sanitation has reached a high technical level; the daily
wastes of millions of people are removed without hazard
to public health. And yet for every difficulty science has
eliminated, the metropolis has created a new and greater
problem in our manner of urban life.

The metropolis lacks nearly all the humanizing
features of early urban life. In the medieval and Renaissance towns, intellectual activity and art were combined

with physical labor; in the metropolis, intellectual activity, art, and physical labor are sharply separated. The civil engineer who designs a structure seldom participates in its construction; his counterpart in the field rarely engages in design. Architects like Frank Lloyd Wright, who concerned himself with nearly every phase of construction, are rarities. Most jobs in the metropolis are sedentary and monotonous. Some of the more rapidly growing occupations require very little mental or physical work; they are mindless as well as sedentary. Work of this kind is typified by the tasks of the billing-machine operator and the dictaphone pool typist, whose principal qualification is the ability to endure an excruciatingly vacuous routine.

The current occupational trend is toward an extreme simplification of the labor process. Work is fragmented, limited, and overspecialized. Modern industry has broken down many highly skilled crafts into repetitive tasks that the worker can perform mechanically, by habit, without losing time either in thinking or in changing tools. Work tends to become sedentary, not because the comfort of the worker is kept in mind, but because any unnecessary movement of the body tends to diminish output by interrupting the smooth, uniform flow of labor. The same trend is evident in intellectual and artistic work, where over-specialization tends to replace creative activity with mechanical operations. While many such jobs allow for considerable individual leeway, progressively fewer faculties are used or developed. In the worst cases, physical work is limited to a few dexterous operations of the fingers, mental work to a few dexterous operations of the mind.

Labor becomes highly intensive. The few faculties that are brought into play are employed at continually higher rates of speed. Work is viewed more as a function of habit than as the function of individual resources and talents whose use requires patience and tolerance. Thus, many jobs not only tend to restrict the use of certain parts of the body, but employ other parts excessively. Forms of work which once mobilized the human organism as a whole are supplanted by occupations that tax the eyes or the nerves. While the mind is dulled and the human musculature becomes flaccid, nerves become overly sensitive and raw. The anxieties and tensions created by intensive, sedentary work are reinforced by an exaggerated responsiveness of the nervous system as a whole.

The metropolis offers very little to counteract the oversimplification of the daily work routine. The urban dweller encounters few changes in color to awaken his visual senses; he receives virtually no respite from the artificial world in which he is immersed during working hours. Areas in which he can walk freely on soil and amid vegetation are disappearing; new dwellings, most of them noteworthy for their lack of architectural inspiration, are encroaching on the last open spaces in American cities. Public parks are likely to be congested during the day, and in the evening they often attract delinquent elements, whose presence discourages the respectable urban dweller from venturing into their precincts. American urban life has retreated indoors. This retreat is due partly to the erosion of human solidarity in large cities, partly to the seductive powers of the mass media. The average urban dweller is likely to pursue the same insensate, sedentary way of life during his leisure time that he follows during his working hours.

Many aspects of metropolitan life, while trivial in themselves, aggravate the effects of urban modes of work. The nervous strain that the city dweller feels at his job begins to gather within him even before he gets to work.

He encounters inconveniences, rudeness, and congestion on public conveyances; he is beleaguered by countless small anxieties, many of which seldom rise to the level of consciousness. An all-pervasive irritation collects within him on his way to work, at work, between working hours, and on the way home. Mechanical noises are everywhere. They invade even the hours of sleep as a result of the growing web of highways that reaches into every part of the city. Advertising media assail the senses with garish images and sounds; their message is crude and elemental, designed to startle and perhaps to shock the viewer into a response. Recreation seldom furnishes the average urban dweller with the experiences denied to him in the daily bustle of life—moments of genuine serenity, silence, and gentle changes of scene. More often than not, urban recreation merely removes him temporarily from the afflictions of his environment without replenishing his reserves. It provides him with surcease from anxiety and nervous strain rather than with restoration of vitality.

Unfortunately, these problems are no longer confined to the city. The metropolis establishes the social standards of the entire country. Owing to its commanding economic and cultural position, it sets the pace of national life and establishes nearly all the criteria of national taste. Many distinctively urban forms of work and play have invaded the most remote rural areas of the United States, where they generate the same stresses in the villager and farmer that they do in the city dweller. The nature of agricultural work, moreover, is changing. As farming becomes increasingly industrialized, diversified physical work is reduced to a minimum by machines and one-crop agriculture. Although the farmer still pursues a less hurried way of life than his urban cousin, he is often beleaguered by even greater economic problems. Both in the city and on the land, a new type of man seems to be emerging. He is a nervous, excitable, and highly strained individual who is burdened by continual personal anxieties and mounting social insecurity.

STRESS AND CHRONIC ILLNESS

WHAT ARE THE EFFECTS of persistent emotional stress on human health?

Fifty years ago this question would have seemed irrelevant to the goals of medical research. The principal illnesses of the day were ascribed to the aging process, to a variety of "mechanical defects," such as blockages and ruptures, to a poor genetic endowment, and to bacterial infection. Germs satisfied the need for precise explanations of disease. They entered the body in a limited number of ways; they could be isolated, cultured, and tested on animals and human volunteers. With further knowledge, it was believed, all the effects produced by harmful bacteria would be understood and eventually controlled by some form of therapy. Emotional stress, on the other hand, was vague. It seemed to represent a generalized response on the part of the body to countless, often intangible stimuli. Although medicine was not unaware of the fact that emotional disturbances influenced the functioning of the heart and gastrointestinal tract, there seemed little reason to believe that stress played a causal role in the major diseases of man.*

* To cite a few exceptions: As early as the 1870's Dr. Jacob Mendes Da Costa described a syndrome which has since acquired the name of cardiac neurosis. Certain digestive disturbances were also recognized as being influenced by the emotional state of a patient, but these were often minor in nature.

As chronic illnesses began to gain in importance, however, it became evident that the earlier approach was inadequate. Many arthritic conditions, for example, could not be explained by infection. Beginning slowly and insidiously, arthritis often produced in the end a hopelessly crippled, bedridden patient who faced a lifetime of pain and inactivity. At the same time, such words as "strain" and "anxiety" began to acquire real physiological meaning, denoting conditions that involved glandular conditions, biochemical changes in tissues, and involuntary activity of the nervous system. It was soon found that these physiological changes could produce or alleviate many of the symptoms associated with the common chronic diseases of our time.

A growing number of physicians now agree that emotional stress is a very important disease-promoting factor. It is safe to say that some disorders, such as peptic ulcers, arise primarily from anxiety and tension. During the latter part of the nineteenth century, peptic ulcers were regarded as a relatively uncommon disorder, and there arose very confused explanations of what caused the illness. Physicians generally believed that it occurred more frequently in women than in men; it was looked upon as a disorder primarily of "chlorotic," or anemic, girls. In the medical textbooks of the day, discussions of peptic ulcers were confined to descriptions of symptoms and dietary therapy. With the passing years, however, the disease became a widespread and serious problem. Today, peptic ulcers afflict about 2½ million Americans; each year nearly 400,000 are disabled for more than a week. Although a case of ulcers may often arouse a great deal of levity, the disease can reach grave proportions. About ten thousand Americans die of peptic ulcers every year. According to data compiled by the U. S. National Health Survey of 1957-9, the overwhelming majority of ulcer victims (73 per cent) are men. More cases appear in the thirty-five-to-forty-four age group—the years of greatest business and vocational activity—than in any other ten-year period of life.

Emotional stress is also deeply implicated in disorders of the blood vessels and the heart. "Physicians have long felt that the rapid pace of modern civilization might somehow be contributing to the development of heart disease," notes a report by the National Heart Institute. "The man who develops coronary artery disease is very frequently a hard-driving individual living in a state of more or less constant tension. In recent years evidence has accumulated that one way in which nervous tension may accelerate the development of coronary artery disease is through an elevation of the [blood] serum cholesterol level."

The evidence is impressive. In 1957, Friedman, Rosenman, and Carroll, of Mount Zion Hospital in San Francisco, began a study of the serum cholesterol level and blood-clotting time in forty male accountants during and after the tax season—sharply contrasting periods of high and low occupational stress. Blood was taken from the accountants twice weekly from January to June, and detailed records were kept of weight, diet, and changing work loads. "When studied individually," the investigators report, "each subject's highest serum cholesterol consistently occurred during severe occupational or other stress, and his lowest at times of minimal stress. The results could not be ascribed to any changes of weight, exercise, or diet. Marked acceleration of blood clotting time consistently occurred at the time of maximum occupational stress, in contrast to normal blood clotting during periods of respite."

Studies of a similar nature have been made of medical students during examination week. In 1958 a report of P. T. Wertlake at the College of Medical Evangelists in Los Angeles showed that the average serum cholesterol level of the students rose 11 per cent during the four-day period in which they took school tests. The investigators found that nearly half of the students responded to the stress situation with increases ranging from 16 to 137 milligram per cent over a mean control level of 213. The serum cholesterol level of one student rose from an average control level of 259 milligram per cent prior to the school examinations to a peak of 536 during one of the examination days—an increase of more than 100 per cent.

It would be wrong to suppose, however, that our knowledge of the link between emotional stress and illness is based entirely on statistical findings. During the past two decades, researchers have discovered a number of the biochemical effects that persistent anxiety produces in the human body. Attention has focused primarily on the adrenal glands, which cap the kidneys. The surface layer, or cortex, of these glands produces a number of highly potent regulatory chemical substances, or hormones. The cortical hormones, or corticoids, help the body to ward off disease and resist the effects of physical damage. A number of adrenal corticoids (aldosterone and DOC, for example) promote inflammation—the heat, swelling, and redness with which tissues react to common injuries. Although inflammation protects the body from bacterial invasion by "walling off" an injured area, the inflammatory process would go too far if it were not for anti-inflammatory corticoids, such as cortisone, which limit the process and prevent it from becoming needlessly widespread. The output of cortisone, in turn, is stimulated by ACTH, a hormone produced by the pituitary gland, situated at the base of the skull. The control of inflammation requires a balanced secretion of ACTH, of the pro-inflammatory corticoids, and of the anti-inflammatory corticoids. If the balance in the secretion of these three types of hormones is altered, the inflammatory process may damage parts of the body.

Secretions of ACTH and the corticoids are influenced by the emotional state of the individual as well as by physical injury. This discovery has aroused strong suspicions that the corticoids and, by inference, persistent nervous strain, anxiety, and emotional conflicts play important roles in the occurrence of certain chronic disorders. In a review of the literature on rheumatoid arthritis and stress, Leon Hellman has suggested that "a more subtle form of stress in the guise of emotional conflicts is implicated in changes of the pituitary-adrenal system so as to render it less responsive or to alter the balance between various adrenal hormones secreted. A patient with rheumatoid arthritis would cure himself if his hypothalamus [a nerve center in the forebrain] and pituitary would interlock to increase the secretion of ACTH . . ." According to Hellman, it is quite possible that the production of ACTH is inhibited by a "neural block" arising from deep-seated emotional conflicts. Both ACTH and cortisone have been used with considerable success in treating arthritic disorders. The hormones alleviate rheumatoid symptoms so dramatically that hopelessly crippled, bedridden arthritics have been restored to almost complete use of their limbs.

The adrenal corticoids, however, influence more than the inflammatory process. They exercise extensive control over the level of minerals and sugar (glucose) in the blood. An imbalance in corticoid secretion is likely to have far-reaching effects on the body's metabolism and on organs that are commonly damaged by metabolic disorders, notably the heart and kidneys. By administering the pro-inflammatory hormone DOC to white Leghorn chicks, for example, Hans Selye and his co-workers at the University of Montreal were able to produce degenerative changes in the kidneys, with ensuing high blood pressure, hardening of the blood vessels, and cardiac disease. During the course of the experiment, the DOC-treated chicks "began to drink much more water than the controls which were not given the hormone, and gradually they developed a kind of dropsy. Their bodies became enormously swollen with fluid accumulations under the skin and they began to breathe with difficulty, gasping for air, just like certain cardiac patients." By degrees, Selye's results and those of other researchers in the field began to include a large number of common chronic illnesses. Pro- and anti-inflammatory corticoids, it was found, seem to play roles of varying importance in diabetes, thyroid disorders, peptic ulcers, and psychic disturbances. The anti-inflammatory corticoids have been very useful in combating many of these illnesses. Cortisone frequently produces striking though temporary remissions in cases of acute leukemia, and the surgical removal of the adrenal glands often inhibits the growth of certain forms of cancer.

Selye has developed a general theory of stress from the data on the interplay of adrenal hormones. Stress consists of the physical changes within an organism which are caused by any environmental stimulus, whether it be heat, cold, infection, or a chemical irritant, and by the emotional disturbances we encounter in man. All living things have an adaptive mechanism that produces changes in the organism in response to changes in its environment. The adrenal corticoids in man and higher animals are essentially chemical agents that compel a living thing to respond internally to external stimuli. Every stimulus, desirable or harmful, produces a general stress reaction. Stress, in effect, is an important part of life.

But stress always results in a certain amount of "wear and tear" on the organism. "Many people believe that, after they have exposed themselves to very stressful activities, a rest can restore them to where they were before," Selye writes. "This is false. Experiments on animals have clearly shown that each exposure leaves an indelible scar, in that it uses up reserves of adaptability which cannot be replaced. It is true that immediately after some harassing experience, rest can restore us almost to the original level of fitness by eliminating acute fatigue. But the emphasis is on the word *almost*. Since we constantly go through periods of stress and rest during life, just a little deficit of adaptation energy every day adds up—it adds up to what we call aging."

No one, to be sure, can eliminate the "wear and tear" of life, but a reasonably clear distinction can be made between the "stress of life" and stress that results in ill health. Stress that results in ill health is severe, persistent, and one-sided. Selye has demonstrated that if stress is too severe, the resistance and life span of the organism are drastically reduced. An experimental rat may adapt itself for a time to a strong irritant, but the adaptation is made at a high price; longevity is decreased and general resistance is seriously impaired. If the animal is exposed to even minor but persistent stress, comparable to the "low-grade" nervous tension and anxiety usually found in modern urban man, it pays a similar price for adaptation. The animal is easily injured by irritants that ordinarily do not produce serious physical damage. The interplay of stress responses is so complex that the reader must turn to Selye's own work, *The Stress of Life,* for a detailed discussion. In nearly all cases of severe or persistent stress, Selye has found evidence of thickened arteries, heart abnormalities, kidney damage, and increased blood pressure.

But Selye's work also demonstrates that stress need not be harmful, provided it is balanced and varied. A sheltered, sedentary life that lacks a variety of stimuli produces an undeveloped, often inadequate stress mechanism as well as an undeveloped personality. A sheltered person has great difficulty in coping with many of the stimuli and irritants inevitably encountered in the normal course of life. If there is any notion that sums up Selye's "stress of life" theory, it is the "pre-scientific" intuition that variety and balance—emotional, physical, and intellectual—are the bases not only for true individuality but for lasting health.

Selye's plea for variety in life, however, rests on a well-thought-out hypothesis. Man, as a complex, multicellular animal, is composed of many organs and systems, each of which bears a different amount of stress. The organs that compose his body do not "wear out" evenly. Death invariably comes "because one vital part has worn out too early in proportion to the rest of the body. . . . The lesson seems to be that, as far as man can regulate his life by voluntary actions, he should seek to equalize stress throughout his being, by what we have called *deviation*, the frequent shifting-over of work from one part to the other. The human body—like the tires on a car, or the rug on a floor—wears longest when it wears evenly. We can do ourselves a great deal of good in this respect by just yielding to our natural cravings for variety in everyday life. We must not forget that the more we vary our actions the less any one part suffers from attrition."

Conceivably, an informed individual can try to cultivate a mature outlook that will lend distance to the petty irritations produced by the urban milieu. If circumstances permit, he can establish a personal regimen of after-work exercise and frequent excursions to the countryside. But on the whole, the metropolis exposes him to limited, intense occupational stimuli that produce an equally limited, intense stress response. A few organs continue to bear nearly the entire burden of daily life. Organs and systems that are not activated by modern forms of work and play are likely to be sheltered by the "conveniences" that the city affords. "One might question whether stress is peculiarly characteristic of our sheltered civilization, with all its comforts and amenities," observe P. C. Constantinides and Niall Carey in a general discussion of Selye's work. "Yet these very protections—modern labor-saving devices, clothing, heating—have rendered us all the more vulnerable and sensitive to the slightest stress. What was a mild stress to our forebears now frequently represents a minor crisis. Moreover, the frustrations and repressions arising from emotional conflicts in the modern world, economic and political insecurity, the drudgery associated with many modern occupations—all these represent stresses as formidable as the most severe physical injuries."

THE PROBLEMS OF OVER-URBANIZATION

A NUMBER OF URBAN PROBLEMS have arisen that no city dweller can hope to solve or even meliorate on his own; they can be solved only by the community as a whole. One such problem, urban air pollution, has become very widespread and constitutes a serious hazard to human health. "Millions of citizens are living in an air ocean that is, on good evidence, unhealthy to breathe," observes Herman E. Hilleboe, New York State Commissioner of Health. "Cities with the heaviest pollution load tend to rank high both in death and incidence rates for a number of diseases. This includes heart disease and cancer, the ranking killers and disablers of our time." Among the new pollutants that will soon be added to our environment, Hilleboe warns, are "by-products from petroleum and from synthetic materials spawned by our fast-growing nuclear technology and from high-energy solid and liquid fuels. We are creating a new environment but we have not as yet done what is necessary to make this environment healthful and habitable for its people. Here again it is difficult to dramatize the matter of air pollution."

The problem has been dramatized by cases in which air pollution reached the proportions of an emergency, comparable in many ways to an epidemic. Until fairly recently, serious cases of air pollution usually occurred in highly industrialized river valleys. Two such cases—one in the Meuse Valley in Belgium in 1930, which claimed sixty lives, and the other in Donora, Pennsylvania, in 1948, which killed twenty people—were due primarily to toxic fumes from metallurgical plants. To some degree, both could be regarded as industrial accidents, which could have been averted if suitable measures had been taken to control the effluents of local mills. A much greater respect for the potentially disastrous consequences of air pollution was created by the smog that descended upon London, a predominantly commercial city, during December 1952. Although the episode was brief, the daily death rate reached very high levels, comparable to those of London's cholera epidemic in 1854 and its influenza epidemic in 1918-19.

At dawn on Friday, December 5, the air in London began to thicken perceptibly. Unusual weather conditions caused a heavy smog of urban pollutants to linger over the city for four days. During the first twenty-four hours the death rate doubled, the total for the day reaching 400. The next day, Saturday, it rose to 600, and on each of the two following days, Sunday and Monday, it soared to 900, although business and industrial activity was suspended on Sunday. On Tuesday, when the smog had already begun to lift, the number of deaths was 800, and the death rate remained high for several weeks thereafter.

The London smog claimed at least 4,000 lives. The majority of deaths occurred among infants and elderly people, but William P. Dowie Logan, Britain's chief medical statistician, emphasizes that "it was by no means confined to the very young or the very old." The death rate in the fifteen-to-forty-four age group increased about 50 per cent. Deaths from coronary heart disease rose from 118 in the seven-day period immediately preceding the incident to 281 in the week that followed it, while deaths from bronchitis soared from 76 to 704, almost a tenfold increase.

The possibility that a lethal smog comparable to the one that descended on London, will develop somewhere in the United States cannot be excluded. If the word "smog" is defined as air pollution that produces haziness in the atmosphere and irritation of the eyes, nose, and throat, then many American communities experience smog. The situation in Los Angeles is notoriously bad; the city is afflicted with fifty to seventy days of smog every year. Smog is found to a lesser extent in New York, Washington, Philadelphia, Boston, and other coastal metropolitan areas of the United States. The differences between smog in England and smog in the United States are due primarily to the differences in the irritants that pervade the air of the two countries. Air pollution in London is caused mainly by the combustion of coal, whereas the principal irritants in Los Angeles are produced by the combustion of petroleum products. Experts have emphasized, however, that "in the London episode the air pollutants, when considered in terms of their human effects, closely resembled those present in the air of many large urban areas. These pollutants were quite similar to those of many other urban areas in that they are irritating to the exposed living membranes (of the eyes, nose, throat and respiratory tract). For example, although Los Angeles air pollution is chemically different from that of London the two resemble each other in their effects on man since each causes irritation of exposed living membranes."

Ordinarily, smog is episodic and localized. In the long run, a more serious problem is posed by persistent, low-grade air pollution, which is often imperceptible to the senses and changes relatively little from day to day. This form of air pollution is very widespread in the United States. Nearly 10,000 communities, containing the overwhelming majority of the American people, have persistent air pollution problems. According to a recent report by the New York State Air Pollution Control Board: "Of the state's 40 communities with populations of more than 25,000, only one had negligible air pollution. The combined survey data show that approximately three-fifths of the communities of 5,000 to 25,000 population, and about one third of those with less than 5,000 people, had major or minor air pollution." A survey of Texas by the U. S. Public Health Service showed that three quarters of the state's communities with populations of more than 10,000 had "objectionable air pollution."

Although patterns of air pollution vary from one community to another, it is generally agreed that the air in nearly all American cities contains a number of highly toxic substances, most of which are waste products of industrial plants, motor vehicles, and heating equipment. The solid particles in an urban atmosphere often include such highly toxic substances as lead, beryllium, and arsenic. Common air-borne gases and vapors include sulfuric-acid mist, sulfur dioxide, carbon monoxide, formaldehyde, oxides of nitrogen, ammonia, and scores of organic vapor contaminants. At least a hundred air pollutants have been identified, and the interaction of gases, vapors, and solid particles in the atmosphere produces many other compounds that have not been chemically analyzed. Several known toxicants that pollute the air are characterized by synergistic activity; they are more toxic together than when each is absorbed individually. For example, an effect that is more than additive is produced by the inhalation of carbon monoxide together with nitrogen oxide, two of the most common pollutants in the urban atmosphere.

The average individual breathes about 16,000 quarts of air daily. If he lives in an urban environment, his lungs receive about four times as many air contaminants as those of a rural dweller. John H. Ludwig, of the U. S. Public Health Service, suggests that repeated exposure to "relatively low levels of air pollution" may be involved in the development of chronic degenerative diseases, including skin and lung cancer, heart and vascular disorders, and chronic bronchitis. During periods when urban air pollution is at its height, the contaminants may worsen existing chronic diseases, especially heart disorders, by interfering with the passage of oxygen through the membranes of the lungs into the blood stream. Certain air pollutants may combine with body proteins to form allergy-inducing, or allergenic, substances and lead to increasing sensitization and allergic reactions.

If the possible consequences of air pollution listed by Ludwig seem to be farfetched, let us enumerate some of the contaminants produced by the automobile, the principal source of air-borne toxicants in large American cities. Nearly 80 per cent of the pollutants that produce smog in Los Angeles come from motor vehicles. In burning 1,000 gallons of fuel, an automobile discharges 17 pounds of sulfur dioxide, about 18 pounds of aldehydes (estimated as formaldehyde), 25 to 75 pounds of oxides of nitrogen (estimated as nitrogen dioxide), 200 to 400 pounds of complex organic compounds, and over 3,000 pounds of carbon monoxide.

Sulfur dioxide is both an irritant and a poison. It is probably a major contributor to the high incidence of chronic bronchitis in England. There is evidence to indicate that a fairly low level of sulfur dioxide—"a level not infrequently found in air"—is sufficient to produce temporary spasms of the smooth muscles in the lungs. In "somewhat higher concentrations," the compound produces severe inflammation and peeling of the respiratory membranes. Formaldehyde is a corrosive poison that not only irritates the respiratory membranes but also affects the central nervous system, and nitrogen dioxide is a highly toxic gas that is extremely dangerous even in such relatively low quantities as 100 parts per million.

Several of the organic compounds produced by the combustion of gasoline and diesel oil are carcinogenic. This has been clearly established by Paul Kotin, of the University of California. When tarry material from the exhausts of motor vehicles was painted on laboratory mice, skin tumors appeared in 50 per cent of the animals. The largest amount of carcinogenic substances, according to Kotin's findings, is produced by slow-running and idling engines—that is, under conditions prevalent in areas with congested traffic (see pages 149-50).

A problem that has been largely ignored in the United States is the danger of chronic carbon monoxide poisoning. Until recently, conventional medical opinion held that carbon monoxide (CO) is rapidly removed from the blood stream. Few physicians regarded the enormous output of the gas by motor vehicles as a danger to public health. According to recent reports, however, carbon monoxide may be retained by the body for relatively long periods of time, perhaps as much as several weeks. The problem has aroused a great deal of concern in Europe, where the conviction is growing that chronic carbon monoxide poisoning is a serious hazard of the automobile era. In the United States, Richard Prindle, of the U. S. Public Health Service, emphasizes that "in a community in which carbon monoxide levels exist, 24 hours a day, seven days a week, for the lifetime of an individual, chronic CO poisoning is a distinct possibility." We need only consider the fact that smoking produces a definite level of carbon monoxide in the blood "to realize that coupling this with frequent, although fluctuating exposures to CO in the ambient air . . . might well lead to serious consequences in a large population."

Another problem that cannot be solved without the co-operation of the entire community is water pollution. Water is a traditional medium for the transmission of germs and toxic substances. During the past three generations vigorous efforts on the part of medical and public health officials have enormously reduced the hazard created by water-borne infectious agents, but today old problems of pollution are beginning to recur and new ones to appear, especially in communities that obtain the greater part of their drinking water from rivers. Although

Americans tend to make a fetish of cleanliness, an appalling amount of untreated or inadequately treated urban sewage is discharged into river water—water which is often taken up again for public consumption by communities downstream. Added to urban sewage are wastes from chemical factories, slaughterhouses, and metallurgical plants. Although sewage and industrial wastes have produced local public health crises in the past, the postwar expansion of cities and metropolitan areas is turning water pollution into a grave national problem, comparable in many respects to that created by urban air pollution.

Attempts by federal, state, and municipal authorities to control the contamination of our water are complicated by frequent changes in the composition of industrial and urban wastes. Today drinking water may contain a wide variety of new bleaches, detergents, petrochemical and metallurgical wastes, insecticides, dyes, and radioactive compounds. Few if any of these contaminants are removed by ordinary methods of water purification. Rolf Eliassen, of the Massachusetts Institute of Technology, points out that the "exotic organic chemicals" discharged by petrochemical plants into streams "are not even detected by present conventional means of water analysis." Neither industry nor pollution-control laboratories have been able to form a reliable picture of the long-range effects of the newer pollutants on public health. "Let us all be honest with ourselves," declares Robert A. Kehoe. "Specifications for human health and welfare, in relation to the common contaminants of many of our sources of water, do not exist, and we shall not be able to deal effectively with this problem of public health until they can be formulated on sound physiological facts."

At the same time, the traditional problem of waterborne infections is gaining greater significance. Many cases of acute illnessess are being attributed to polluted drinking water. To cite a few examples: In 1957 the number of cases of infectious hepatitis began to increase markedly in Nebraska. The disease, an acute inflammation of the liver, was found predominantly in the eastern part of the state. The outbreaks occurred primarily in urban communities that obtain their drinking water from the highly polluted Missouri River. Although most public health officials tend to be extremely cautious in their comments, Nebraskan authorities made no attempt to conceal their suspicion that the increase in hepatitis cases was due to drinking water contaminated by sewage from upstream communities. Similar explanations have been given for polio epidemics in Salt Lake City and in Edmonton, capital of the Canadian province of Alberta.* Both diseases are caused by viruses that are found in human feces and sewage.

True, water-borne diseases and, in some communities, urban air pollution have been more serious in the past than they are today. In 1832, Asiatic cholera spread from Quebec to New York City, where it claimed thousands of lives. Cholera persisted in the city for decades before it was eradicated. Typhoid fever, another water-borne disease, was found everywhere during the last century. Owing to improved methods of public sanitation, the incidence of the disease is now negligible. Similarly, many of the worst pockets of urban air pollution are being "cleared up," to the extent of eliminating some of the dense soot and smoke. The cloud of industrial soot that began to descend on Pittsburgh as early as the 1860's

---

* Much of the evidence pointing to polluted water as the cause of these outbreaks is circumstantial, but there is no longer any doubt that hepatitis can be communicated by water as well as by personal contact. The Edmonton outbreak suggests that poliomyelitis can also be transmitted by water. Edmonton obtains its drinking water from the Saskatchewan River and the epidemic could be related to a failure of the sewage system at a town upstream.

has been lifted. Although Pittsburgh does not enjoy pure air, a reduction has been achieved in the more offensive pollutants that once filled the city's atmosphere. Air pollution programs have gained ground primarily against the smoke and grime of the old Industrial Revolution, just as social reform has scored its greatest triumphs over illiteracy and child labor.

Since World War II, however, there has been a new industrial revolution, and the problems of urban life have acquired new dimensions. On the one hand, the sources of urban pollution have increased in number and variety; many pollutants, such as those produced by the automobile, are difficult to manage, even where everyone is willing to co-operate on the problem. On the other hand, metropolitan regions are being burdened beyond their capacity to cope with air pollutants and to meet the need for clean water. Their waterways and atmosphere are expected to absorb a staggering quantity of waste products from industrial plants, homes, and vehicles. Currently the United States must dispose of over 18 billion pounds of sewage solids every year, an increase of 70 per cent in the past two decades. The water table in many areas of the United States is being lowered by the voracious demands of highly concentrated populations and expanding industries. At the same time that the number of pollutants has increased, the ecological preconditions for wholesome air and plentiful water are being undermined. A major disequilibrium is arising between town and country, industry and the biotic environment, and population and regional resources.

Rene Dubos, of the Rockefeller Institute for Medical Research, places smog among the major environmental factors that have unleashed the "Apocalyptic horsemen" of modern disease. According to Dubos, St. John the Divine's vision on the isle of Patmos is symbolic of pres-

ent-day urban and industrial life. The first horsemen of
the Apocalypse to be seen by the saint were Famine and
Pestilence. "Then another, even more terrifying visitation
was sent by the angered Deity," Dubos recalls. "After the
fifth angel had sounded his trumpet he opened the bottomless pit and 'there arose a smoke out of the pit, as the
smoke of a great furnace; and the sun and the air were
darkened by reason of the smoke of the pit.' And out of
the bottomless pit came the scorpions that did not kill
men but tormented them for five months before final
destruction came 'by the fire, and by the smoke and by
the brimstone.' The time of fulfillment of the Apocalypse
may not be far off."

Dubos is not being overly dramatic. We are producing a new spectrum of environmental hazards whose full
effects still await the passage of time. The trends are not
encouraging. "Many diseases that are thought to be associated with, or caused by, air pollution have been
increasing over the years," Prindle writes. "Included
amongst these are the respiratory cancers, emphysema,
chronic bronchitis, and cor pulmonale.* If air pollution
continues to increase, one can only conjecture that this
rising incidence of disease will continue and that the
effect upon the health of the nation—and over the tech-
nologically-expanding world—may be severely augmented.
The overall effect of air pollution on the economy, the
health, and the welfare of the people may become a
disaster."

The effects of air pollution on public health will be

---

* Emphysema is a pulmonary disorder that often leads to cor
pulmonale, a common form of heart disease. Emphysema has become a major disease in London, ranking third (following heart
diseases and cancer) as a cause of death among middle-aged
males. The increase in emphysema cases, both in London and
Los Angeles, is attributed by many medical authorities to air pollution.

difficult to judge for many years to come. A large number of adults straddle two worlds. They were born and raised in communities that have only recently acquired the features of metropolitan life. The early years of their lives were spent in the pre-nuclear age. But it is difficult to ignore the portents found in the high incidence of chronic diseases in all age groups of the population. Without a basic solution to the problems of urban life, Dubos's apprehension may prove to be amply justified.

CHAPTER FOUR

The Problem of Chemicals in Food

THE CONSUMER AND COMMERCIAL FOODS

WITH THE RISE of an urbanized society, the production of food becomes a complex industrial operation. In contrast with earlier times, when very few changes were made in the appearance or the constituents of food, much of the food consumed in the United States is highly processed. Allen B. Paul, of the Brookings Institution, and Lorenzo B. Mann, of the Farmer Cooperative Service, have summed up the change as follows: "Our grandparents used for baking about four-fifths of the flour milled in this country. They churned almost all the butter Americans ate. They killed and prepared much of the meat eaten. They made their own soups, sausage, salad dressing, clothing and countless other items. Such tasks, which a generation ago were part of farm and home life, have been taken over by commercial factories, 85,000 of them." Of the 85,000 factories cited by Paul and Mann, nearly half were food-processing plants.

It is hardly necessary to emphasize the fact that advances in food technology and methods of transportation have given us many advantages. A large number of seasonal fruits and vegetables are now available throughout the year in canned and frozen form. Foods are generally cleaner than they were a half century ago. Processed foods have enormously reduced the homemaker's burden. Many vegetables, fruits, and meats are shredded, eviscerated, mixed, creamed, cooked, baked, or fried before they reach the kitchen. The homemaker often needs little more than a can opener, a few utensils, and a stove to serve meals that required elaborate preparation and hours of work a generation or two ago.

But the shift from home-prepared to processed foods has not been an absolute gain. Although very little was known about human nutrition a few generations ago, our forebears could make use of what knowledge they had in growing and preparing their own foods. Today the situation is different. A great deal has been learned about the nutrients required for human health, but the cultivation, storage, refining, and, in large part, the preparation of food is no longer controlled by the consumer. These tasks have been taken over by the food industry. In the absence of a nation-wide food-grading program that would compel processors to disclose the nutritive values of food items, the housewife's attempt to plan a healthful diet depends to a great extent upon chance. The nutritive quality of a given food may vary enormously. The variation may be due to the type of seed that the farmer plants, the methods employed in food cultivation and food processing, or the length of time the food is stored.

For example: Nutritionists, in analyzing thirty-one strains of cabbage, found that the ascorbic-acid, or vitamin-C, content varied as much as 350 per cent, while the amount of carotene in different varieties of sweet potatoes has been found to range from zero to 7.2 milligrams per cent. A threefold difference was discovered in the niacin content of forty-six strains of sweet corn. Large variations in nutritive value have been found among different varieties of apples, peas, wheat, onions, and many other crops. The fact that a given variety attains great size does not necessarily mean that it is nutritious. The very opposite may be true. Small cabbages, tomatoes, and onions, for example, contain more vitamin C than those of greater size. Size, appearance, color, and texture are often very poor criteria for judging the nutritive content of a food. Generally, plant breeders are interested in developing varieties of vegetables and fruits that have an attractive appearance, yield more bushels to the acre, are more resistant to disease, and withstand storage and shipment. "It is now realized that in the development of these commercially improved varieties by genetic selection the nutrient content is often decreased," notes Robert S. Harris, of the Massachusetts Institute of Technology. "If the plant breeder were to collaborate with a food analysis laboratory, he could develop commercially improved varieties which are also superior in nutrient content." *

Foods may lose much of their nutritive value when they are heated (blanched) prior to canning or freezing.

* It is quite doubtful, however, whether improvements in the nutritive quality of vegetables and fruits depend exclusively on genetic selection (as Harris seems to believe). The plant environment, notably the condition and fertility of the soil, is a factor of decisive importance.

If the processor follows a good blanching procedure, vegetables will retain most of their ascorbic acid and vitamin B. But if the procedure is poor, the losses may be enormous. Losses may run as high as 30 per cent of the riboflavin in green beans, 37 per cent of the naicin in spinach, 40 per cent of the ascorbic acid in peas, and 64 per cent of the thiamine in lima beans. "Blanching procedures are not standardized," Mildred M. Boggs and Clyde L. Rasmussen observe. "Some processors have a leaching loss of 5 to 10 per cent of each water-soluble vitamin or other constituents. Others have losses of 40 to 50 per cent—or even higher with the same food."

A substantial loss of nutrients takes place when wheat is refined into flour for white bread. "Even with 4 per cent milk solids in the white enriched bread," Bogert notes, "it is still not quite up to the content of whole wheat bread in protein, calcium, iron, thiamine and niacin, while the whole grain breads contain other B complex vitamins not added in the enrichment of white flour." If a product is stored too long, it may lose a substantial amount of thiamine. "Pork luncheon," for example, may lose 20 per cent of its thiamine in the can while standing on the retailer's shelf for three months. After six months the loss may be as high as 30 per cent.

Many of these problems could be solved by establishing a compulsory system of grade labeling for processed foods based on their nutritive constituents. The grade markings that currently appear on labels are often meaningless from a nutritional point of view. For the most part, they indicate the food's size, appearance, and taste, not its nutritive value. But the food industry has been adamantly opposed to any kind of compulsory grade labeling. Jesse V. Coles, professor of home economics at the University of California, observes that "practically all, if not all, manufacturers, processors, and distributors are opposed to compulsory grade labeling." In the thirties the food industry defeated attempts to provide for grade labeling in the N.R.A. fair competition codes; it was bitterly opposed to the inclusion of standards of food quality in the food and drug legislation enacted by Congress in 1938; and it successfully blocked efforts to link price regulations with food quality in wartime anti-inflationary laws.

In the absence of a meaningful system of grade labeling, the homemaker is surrounded by nutritional anarchy. Her choice of a product is often governed by its appearance; if it is packaged, she is likely to choose a well-advertised brand or one that is attractively wrapped. Her difficulties are complicated by the fact that many processors color the food she sees and use chemicals to soften the refined products she touches. Preservatives are often added to foods to permit longer storage, and synthetic flavoring matter is put into many processed foods to enhance their taste. And even in those cases in which appearance, taste, and softness are true indications of superior nutritional quality, the processor frequently uses a large variety of chemicals to make an inferior, stale, or overly refined product seem high in quality.

Aside from the deception they practice on the consumer, many of the chemicals added to foods are known to be active toxicants. Presumably they are "safe under the conditions of their intended use," to borrow a phrase formulated by the Food and Drug Administration, but the word "safe" does not mean that the chemicals do no damage. In view of the fact that they are harmful even in relatively small quantities, it is likely that toxicants in foods inflict a certain amount of damage on nearly all animal organisms, including man. Another group of food additives is enveloped in an air of biochemical mystery; very little is known about how they react during animal metabolism. Many additives are chemically unique or "exotic." Until they were developed by chemists, the compounds never appeared in foods, and their long-range effects on the human body have yet to be determined.

The overwhelming majority of people in the United States derive their nourishment from commercial foods. If a harmful chemical finds its way into a popular food, many individuals are likely to be affected. These individuals differ in age, state of health, genetic endowment, environmental background, and susceptibility to the toxicity of the chemical. Some individuals may be more vulnerable to the toxicant than others, although they may never show any symptoms of acute illness.* The research devoted to chemicals in foods seldom goes beyond the effects they produce in laboratory animals. A chemical additive is tested on rats and dogs for about two years. If the chemical causes no apparent damage to tissues and organs, it may be used in food. If it is obviously toxic "under the conditions of its intended use," it will be rejected. But laboratory animals are not men. Their physiology is different from that of human beings and they are unable to communicate important reactions that may well escape the notice of the researcher. Although experiments on rats, dogs, and even monkeys are useful in forewarning man against harmful substances, they do not supply

* There have been cases, however, in which hundreds and even thousands of people suffered acute disorders caused by chemical additives in commercial foods. According to newspaper accounts, as recently as 1960 nearly 100,000 people in the Netherlands were poisoned by a chemical emulsifier that had been added to a popular margarine. The margarine was manufactured by one of the most reputable food processors in Europe. The emulsifier produced an eczema-like rash on many parts of the body and temperatures as high as 106 degrees. At least two deaths were attributed to the emulsifier. About 5 million packages of margarine had been distributed to retailers before the effects of the additive were discovered.

conclusive evidence that chemicals which cause no apparent damage to animals are harmless to man.

Evidence that a chemical is harmful may well appear years after it has been permitted in foods. The use of additives regarded as safe only a decade or two ago has been forbidden because later, more exacting studies showed that these chemicals have toxic properties. According to *Consumer Reports,* coal-tar dyes were certified by the Food and Drug Administration for use as food colors "on the basis of hasty, old-fashioned, and otherwise inadequate testing, and recent advances in research methodology have led to the conclusion that the safety of most of them is unknown. Since 1945, when the FDA began to apply modern methods of study and research to certifiable dyes, 15 food dyes have been re-examined for toxic, carcinogenic or allergenic properties. Only one of these, Yellow No. 5 (used to color candies, icings, and pie-fillings, for example) has been conclusively shown to be harmless. Last year [1955], Orange No. 1, Orange No. 2, and Red No. 32 were decertified as too toxic for use in foods. The FDA announcement said that 'while manufacturers will no longer label and sell these three colors for use, they may label and sell them for external drug and cosmetic use.' Orange No. 1 had been widely used in candy, cakes, cookies, carbonated beverages, desserts, and such meat products as frankfurters. Orange No. 2 and Red No. 32 were used to color the outer skin of oranges, and during the Christmas season last year, some 150 children were made ill in California as a result of eating popcorn colored with Red No. 32."

Whether a food additive is classified as harmful or not depends not only upon laboratory techniques but on the standards of the researcher. Every investigator is confronted with the following questions: How thoroughly should the chemical be studied? On how many species?

What constitutes reasonable evidence that a chemical additive is harmless to man? In hearings before the Delaney Committee more than a decade ago, many conflicting answers were given to these questions. Some eminent researchers advanced the view that tests should be conducted through the whole life span of many animal species, while others seemed to be satisfied with limited experiments on rats. The generally accepted criteria for evaluating the toxicity of food additives represent an unstable compromise between widely divergent scientific views and are subject to serious challenge.

While disputes over the adequacy of current testing standards continue, the problem of chemical additives in food becomes greater with every passing year. Chemicals are used in nearly every phase of the production, storage, and merchandising of food. It is difficult to find a single commercial food that has not been exposed to a chemical compound at some stage of cultivation or processing. Many foods accumulate a large number of residues and additives as they travel from the farm through the processing plant to the retail outlet. Grain, for example, is dusted repeatedly with insecticides and fungicides and then treated with fumigants during storage. At the processing stage, chemicals are added to facilitate handling and to improve the consistency of the flour. The flour is bleached and treated with preservatives. The final product may be colored and wrapped in chemically treated paper that sometimes transfers undesirable substances to the food. Are all of these chemicals indispensable to an ample supply of food? Do any of them constitute hazards to public health? At a time when the number of chemicals in our food is reaching staggering proportions, these questions require considered replies.

CHEMICALS IN AGRICULTURE

THE CLAIM IS OFTEN MADE that without chemicals to protect our orchards and fields from pests, we could not possibly have a modern, productive system of agriculture. "There is abundant evidence that our fruit, vegetables and many other staple crops cannot be produced economically, efficiently, and in an adequate volume without chemical protection from insects, plant diseases, weeds, and other pests," observes George C. Decker, a noted American entomologist. "To deny agriculture the use of these chemical tools would be to jeopardize our agricultural economy and an adequate, well-balanced food supply for the American public. Uninhibited insects and plant diseases would largely eliminate the commercial production of such crops as apples, peaches, citrus fruits, tomatoes, and potatoes, to mention only a few, and would drastically curtail the production of many other major crops."

Although no one would want to jeopardize our agricultural economy, still less deny the American people a well-balanced diet, a great deal of public and professional concern has been aroused by the presence of pesticidal residues in food. An insecticide should be "used as a stiletto rather than a scythe," A. W. A. Brown writes. "Ideally it should be employed to punch a particular hole in the food chain, which, if it cannot be filled in by [other species in the] neighboring elements of the biota, at least should be done at such a time of season that it does not seriously disturb the biota." In practice, the trend has gone in the opposite direction. Insecticides are not only becoming more lethal; they are being used with less and less discrimination. Aside from the ecological implications of this trend, the growing toxicity and variety of insecticidal residues in food have become one of the major health problems of our time.

The large-scale application of insecticides to field crops did not get under way until the 1860's, when a large number of American farmers began to use paris green (copper acetoarsenite) against the Colorado potato beetle. The effectiveness of this insecticide encouraged chemists to develop a variety of other formulas. Most of the new insecticides were inorganic compounds—preparations of arsenic, mercury, and sulfur—which normally remained on the crop after harvesting. The residues ranged in amount from mere traces to quantities large enough to be hazardous to the consumer. As early as 1919 the Boston Board of Health condemned shipments of western pears because of excessive arsenic residue, and six years later British health authorities raised strong objections to the amount of arsenic found on imported American apples. Finally, federal officials placed limits on the amount of arsenic that could be allowed to remain on commercial apples and pears. Ironically, for a brief period the original limits, or tolerances, for food sold to domestic consumers were two and a half times higher than those established for apples exported to Europe.

Although the prewar era of inorganic insecticides has been described as pristine in comparison with the present era of organic preparations, the situation was far from ideal. In the 1930's one of the most widely used inorganic compounds, lead arsenate, combined a suspected carcinogen (arsenic) with a cumulative poison (lead). Calcium arsenate seriously damaged the soil, especially soils low in humus. Many areas of Washington and South Carolina were rendered unproductive as a result of being dusted with large amounts of arsenicals.

Harmful as they are, however, prior to 1945 inorganic insecticides were employed in relatively modest quantities and in a limited variety. The most lethal preparations were used primarily for agricultural purposes, and the greater part of the residue could be removed from the surface of the crops by careful washing.

After World War II, the insecticide problem acquired entirely new dimensions. The total quantity of insecticides used prior to the war was but a fraction of the amount employed in the mid-1950's. Annual domestic sales of pesticides (primarily insecticides) increased more than sevenfold between 1940 and 1956. Inorganic insecticides, though still in use, declined markedly in importance; they were supplanted for the most part by a whole new group of organic preparations. Of these the best known is DDT, a chlorinated hydrocarbon; it was synthesized as early as 1874, but it remained a little-known chemical compound until the late 1930's, when the Swiss chemist Paul Müller discovered its insecticidal properties. The American armed forces began using it in 1943, a year after the first small quantities had been shipped to the United States for experimental purposes. While the war was still in progress, A. P. Dupire in France and F. J. Thomas in England began to work with benzene hexachloride (BHC), another chlorinated hydrocarbon that had been synthesized in the last century. The research of Thomas and his colleagues led to the discovery of the insecticidal properties of lindane, a form of BHC. Significant work was also being done in Germany during this period. Shortly before the war, Gerhard Schrader, while engaged in research on poison gases, discovered a series of extremely lethal organic phosphates, from which parathion, malathion, and other now familiar preparations were developed. The list continued to grow until an impressive number of chlorinated hydrocarbons and organic phosphates were available for use on farms and in gardens, warehouses, stores, and homes.

In retrospect, the carelessness with which some of these insecticides were delivered to the public is incredible. The chemical behavior of the chlorinated hydrocarbons inside the human body is still unknown, although it has been determined that both the chlorinated hydrocarbons and the organic phosphates are powerful nerve toxicants. The organic phosphates are known to inactivate the enzyme cholinesterase, which participates in the chemical control of nerve impulses.* Solutions of organic insecticides are absorbed through the skin as well as the lungs and digestive tract. The skin does not offer an effective barrier to the entry of these toxicants when they are used in liquid form. The younger an organism, the more easily it is poisoned. Both groups of insecticides produce effects in warm-blooded animals very similar to those they produce in insects. Farm animals poisoned by DDT and other chlorinated hydrocarbons first become restless and excitable; the next stage is characterized by twitching, spasms, and, finally, convulsions. Animals poisoned by the organic phosphates usually die of respiratory failure, but in these cases, too, convulsions have been known to occur.

Fortunately, DDT, the first of the new organic insecticides to be widely used, is one of the milder chlorinated hydrocarbons. The compound began to reach

* Until recently, virtually nothing was known about the effects of extended exposure to low doses of organic phosphates, and it was generally assumed that there were no long-term effects at all. In June 1961, however, S. Gershon and F. H. Shaw, of the University of Melbourne, reported that schizophrenic and depressive reactions, with severe impairment of memory and difficulty in concentrating, were found in sixteen individuals who had been exposed to organic phosphates for one and a half to ten years.

American farms in 1945. As test samples of DDT had arrived in the United States only three years earlier, American research on the compound up to that time had been necessarily limited. Some of its more disquieting features were still under study when many Americans began using it with reckless abandon as a "magic bullet" against insect pests. At this stage, very little was known about the way the human body reacts to DDT, the possibility of chronic toxicity, the existence of the indirect routes by which DDT enters the human body, and DDT's stability under varying agricultural conditions. By 1950, when a number of these questions had been answered, it had become evident that although the insecticide is certainly a "magic bullet," the target toward which it is traveling is very much in doubt.

It was found that DDT tends to concentrate heavily in fat. A relatively low dietary intake of the insecticide is magnified from six to twenty-eight times in the fat deposits of the body. According to A. J. Lehman, of the F.D.A., the continual ingestion of as little as 5 parts per million (ppm) of DDT in the diet produces "definite though minimal liver damage" in rats. Such an intake is not likely to be uncommon in the United States. The F.D.A. has placed a residue tolerance of 7 parts per million of DDT on nearly every fruit, vegetable, and portion of animal fat that reaches the American dinner table. But the agency does not know how many farmers are honoring these tolerances. As recently as December 1959, F.D.A. Commissioner George P. Larrick confessed that economic incentives to use chemicals in agriculture are so compelling that his organization "can hardly be expected to control the problem adequately."

The reputation of DDT suffered its first blow only two years after the end of the war, As early as 1947, Italian entomologists noted that DDT-resistant flies were appearing in many parts of Italy. Similar reports began to come from California and other areas in the United States. By 1950, American surveys had shown that previously susceptible strains of flies "were becoming resistant to DDT over a period of 2 or 3 years." Entomologists and public health workers were still hopeful that the malaria-carrying mosquito would continue to succumb to DDT, but this insect also developed DDT-resistant strains. As the number of resistant insects began to multiply, attention shifted to more lethal preparations, such as chlordane, dieldrin, and the organic phosphates.

Chlordane and the dieldrin-aldrin group of preparations are highly toxic chlorinated hydrocarbons. A portion of the testimony and data that the Delaney Committee received on chlordane is summarized in its report as follows: "The Director of the Division of Pharmacology of the Food and Drug Administration [A. J. Lehman] testified that from a chronic viewpoint chlordane is four to five times more toxic than DDT, and that he would hesitate to eat food that had any [chlordane] residue on it whatever. He stated that chlordane has no place in the food industry where even the remotest opportunity for contamination exists, and that it should not be used even as a household spray or in floor waxes." Later experimental work showed that chlordane, when fed to rats, has about twice the chronic toxicity of DDT; the insecticide produces detectable liver damage when ingested in amounts as low as 2½ parts per million.

Dieldrin and aldrin, according to Lehman, create a danger of chronic toxicity that "may be similar" to that posed by chlordane. These insecticides have the "rather rare property of being more toxic by skin absorption than by oral ingestion, the ratio being about 10:1. To state this another way, dieldrin and aldrin are approximately 10 times more poisonous when applied to the skin than when swallowed. . . . Neither of these compounds is irritating to the skin in low concentrations so that the individual has no warning of skin contact."

The F.D.A. permits residues of chlordane, dieldrin, and aldrin on nearly all the vegetables and fruits sold to American consumers. In view of current spraying practices, it is not unusual for foods to accumulate residues of several chlorinated hydrocarbons. The fact that the various insecticides have different chemical properties is small reason for comfort. "Studies in our laboratories have shown that when low concentrations of several insecticides are fed to rats the effect is additive," Lehman writes. "For example, when 2 ppm each of DDT, chlordane, lindane, toxaphene, and methoxychlor, making a total of 10 ppm of chlorinated hydrocarbons, are added to the diet of rats, liver damage results. With the possible exception of chlordane, none of the insecticides listed, when fed individually at 2 ppm, would injure the liver, but in their combination their effect is additive."

Where do we stand today in our chemical war against the insect world? Although partial control has been achieved over some carriers of disease, and other pests are no longer the nuisance they once were, the basic problems of insect infestation remain unsolved. Herbert F. Schoof observes that "man's insect enemies are adapting to successful coexistence with pesticides almost as rapidly as new technics and toxicants are produced." We are paying a heavy price for our questionable gains against agricultural pests. A larger quantity of insecticides is required almost every year. The production of DDT in the United States nearly doubled between 1950, when the compound was no longer a novelty, and 1958. Nearly 100 million pounds of aldrin, chlordane, dieldrin, endrin, heptachlor, and toxaphene—chemicals virtually unknown to farmers in the 1940's—were produced in 1958. Approximately 3 billion pounds of pesticides, including herbicides, fungicides, and fumigants, are produced annually in the United States. "The pesticide industry is growing by leaps and bounds and entomologists predict, and chemical manufacturers hope for, a fourfold expansion in use of pesticides during the next ten to fifteen years," observes Clarence Cottam, of the Welder Wildlife Foundation. "Today, well over 12,500 brandname formulations and more than 200 basic control compounds are on the market. Most of the currently used pesticides were unknown even ten years ago. Furthermore, and contrary to the public interest, most new pesticides are decidedly more toxic, generally more stable, and less specific in effect than those of but a few years back."

The postwar era also witnessed the introduction of highly potent chemical agents for increasing the weight of livestock. In 1947 the F.D.A. approved the use of stilbestrol pellets for "tenderizing" the meat of poultry. Stilbestrol, a synthetically prepared drug, causes bodily changes that are identical with those produced by certain female sex hormones (estrogens). The drug was approved for use with the understanding that poultrymen would implant a single pellet in the upper region of the chicken's neck about a month or two before marketing. Presumably this period was sufficient for the complete absorption of the chemical, so that no residues would be left in the flesh of the bird. Male birds treated with stilbestrol undergo radical physiological changes; their reproductive organs, combs, and wattles shrivel, and they lose all inclination to crow or fight. The drug tends to cause substantial increases in weight in both sexes, producing plump birds with skin that is noticeably smooth in texture.

Careful investigation has shown that stilbestrol increases the over-all fat content of chickens by 40 per cent. In the hearings before the Delaney Committee, Robert K. Enders, professor of zoology at Swarthmore College, expressed his agreement "with those endocrinologists who say that the use of the drug to fatten poultry is an economic fraud. Chicken feed is not saved; it is merely turned into fat instead of protein. Fat is abundant in the American diet so more is undesirable. Protein is what one wants from poultry. By their own admission it is the improvement in appearance and increase in fat that makes it more profitable to the poultryman to use the drug. This fat is of very doubtful value and is in no way the dietary equal of the protein that the consumer thinks he is paying for."

By the late 1950's approximately 100 million hormone-treated fowl were being marketed annually to American consumers. In a number of limited surveys, the F.D.A. found that stilbestrol pellets often remained in the necks of poultry until after the birds had reached wholesale outlets; the pellets were not completely absorbed. Stilbestrol was detected in the edible tissues of hormone-treated fowl even after the heads and necks had been removed. Finally, in December 1959, the F.D.A. announced that, on its recommendation, the poultry industry had agreed to discontinue the use of the synthetic estrogen. It is doubtful whether either the F.D.A. or the poultry industry had very much choice. Stilbestrol is suspected of being a cancer-promoting drug, and recent federal legislation specifically prohibits the presence of carcinogenic additives in food. Pellets of stilbestrol are still implanted in the ears of cattle, however, and the drug is widely used as a supplement to the feed of steers and sheep. The official opinion today is that no residues of the drug will remain in large animals if breeders obey F.D.A. regulations, but the evidence to support this opinion is open to question (see pages 140-1).

The use of synthetic estrogens in livestock management was soon followed by the addition of antibiotics to feed, a technique that dramatically accelerates the growth of domestic animals. Although there is no evidence that antibiotics affect the nutritive quality of meat, research conducted by the F.D.A. showed that chlortetracycline and penicillin could be detected in the blood, tissues, and eggs of chickens given feed containing as little as 50 parts per million of the drugs. This quantity does not exceed the limits established by the F.D.A. for antibiotics in feed. According to William A. Randall, of the F.D.A.'s Division of Antibiotics, the "small amounts found in chicken tissue were destroyed following frying. Furthermore, when the antibiotic-containing feed was withdrawn and normal feeding begun the antibiotic disappeared from the tissue or eggs within a few days. After hard-boiling eggs containing antibiotics, no activity could be detected in the great majority of those tested."

But we should place the emphasis where it properly belongs. Antibiotics could be detected even in eggs that were hard-boiled, and residues were found in the tissues and eggs of chickens after normal feeding was restored. Accordingly, current F.D.A. regulations prohibit the use of antibiotics in the feed of egg-laying hens and require that, in the case of poultry destined for human consumption, normal feeding be restored four days prior to slaughtering. "It may well be in the public interest to reserve this valuable class of drugs for the purpose for which they were originally developed," Randall concludes, "that is, the prevention and treatment of disease."

This conclusion is not without merit. Many farmers pay very little attention to the F.D.A.'s regulations, and nearly all farmers ignore them at one time or another. The situation is similar to that faced by the police in trying to keep motorists from speeding; almost everyone

occasionally exceeds the speed limit. But in the case of the
F.D.A. regulations, the violator's chances of being caught
are infinitesimal in comparison with those of the speeder.
Although its inspection program is totally inadequate to
cope with the problem of chemicals in food, the F.D.A.
has already discovered violations of its regulations on
feed supplemented with arsenic compounds, another
widely used promoter of growth. "A very preliminary survey made some time ago by the Food and Drug Administration indicated that some poultry raisers are not with-
holding arsenic-containing feeds from their flocks 5 days
before slaughter," complained Arthur S. Flemming, former Secretary of Health, Education, and Welfare, "and
we have information that in some parts of the country,
hog raisers maintain their animals on arsenic-containing
feed within the 5-day period that the arsenic is supposed
to be withheld. It is evident that such disregard for safe
use could lead to added arsenic residues in poultry and
pork on the retail market and thus could frustrate the
public health safeguards upon which the original ap-
provals were granted."

Antibiotics are dangerous food additives. The sensitivity of many persons to penicillin has reached a point
where a therapeutic dose of the drug can be expected to
claim their lives. Such individuals are increasing in number with every passing year. Cases have already been
reported in which penicillin used to treat infections in
dairy cattle entered the milk supply in sufficient quantities
to cause severe reactions in human consumers. According
to Murray C. Zimmerman, of the University of Southern
California, data on milk contamination suggest that a
person who drinks two quarts of milk every day "could
ingest over 1,000 units of penicillin daily. The fact that
penicillin 'naturally' present in milk has not previously
been proved to cause allergic reactions is outweighed by

the fact that *this is almost a billion times more penicillin than has previously been shown necessary to provoke reactions.* Coleman and Siegel reported a patient with a reaction on passive transfer to 0.00001 units of penicillin. Bierlein's patient went into shock when skin-tested with 0.000003 units of penicillin." Zimmerman then proceeds to discuss detailed case histories of four patients whose reaction to penicillin could be traced with reasonable certainty to the consumption of dairy products.

It is quite conceivable that the extensive use of antibiotics in agriculture will slowly turn our domestic animals into a major reservoir of antibiotic-resistant bacteria. This represents a problem fraught with incalculable dangers to public health. Feed supplemented with tetracycline, for example, has already produced resistant strains of *Bacterium coli* and *Clostridium perfigens.* Both bacteria typically inhabit man's alimentary tract, but under certain circumstances they behave as disease-causing organisms. "Examination of pigs and poultry kept on many different farms showed that the *B. coli* in the feces of tetracycline-fed animals were predominantly tetracycline-resistant," observes H. William Smith, of the Animal Health Trust in Sussex, England, "while those in the feces of animals on farms where tetracycline feeding was not practiced were predominantly tetracycline-sensitive. In some herds in which tetracycline feeding was just being introduced it was possible to trace the changes of the *B. coli* fecal flora from tetracycline-sensitive to tetracycline-resistant." Smith notes that similar changes could be traced in the case of *Clostridium perfigens.*

The use of shotgun methods to treat or forestall udder infections in cattle with penicillin has almost certainly increased the propagation of resistant strains of *Staphylococcus aureus,* the principal culprit in the common "staph infection" and the direct cause of grave, often fatal cases of pneumonia. Smith notes that the proportion of penicillin-resistant *Staphylococcus aureus* cultures isolated from herd samples of milk in Britain "had increased from 11% in 1954 to 47% in 1956." Two bacteriologists of the Canadian Food and Drug Directorate, F. S. Thatcher and W. Simon, in analyzing cheese that had been purchased in retail outlets, found substantially more penicillin-resistant staphylococci "than would be expected in a normal population not exposed to antibiotic therapy. . . . With regard to the streptococci recovered from cheese our results show a close approximation to the degree of resistance to penicillin found among comparable species isolated from hospital patients."

Thatcher and Simon conclude their report with the warning that "where penicillin or other antibiotics are used with dairy cattle, the survival of resistant organisms may lead to widespread distribution of resistant strains into the homes of the general populace, since staphylococci and streptococci, often in large numbers, are of common occurrence in cheese. Foods so contaminated may well contribute to the severity of the problem arising from infections in man with resistant strains without the patients having received prior antibiotic therapy or without having been exposed to endemic infections within hospitals."

But in the United States this is no longer merely a potential hazard. Already there have been two localized epidemics of "staph infections" that have been attributed to contact with cattle. During 1956 and 1957 about 36 per cent of the senior students and 26 per cent of the faculty at the Veterinary School of the University of Pennsylvania contracted "staph infections." In 1958 another epidemic of the infections occurred among 44 per cent of the senior students at the Colorado State University

College of Veterinary Medicine. There is good reason to believe that, in both cases, animals handled by the students had become a reservoir of antibiotic-resistant staphylococci.

The current trends in agriculture reflect a shocking indifference to the long-term health of our population. By recklessly overcommitting ourselves to the use of chemicals in the growing of our food, we have turned highly potent toxicants and drugs, which we would be justified in using only on a limited scale or in exceptional circumstances, into the foundations of our agriculture. These foundations are extremely unstable and the edifice we are trying to construct may prove to be a trap rather than a habitable dwelling. Insecticides commonly aggravate the very problems they are meant to solve. The ecological difficulties they create lead to the use of increasingly toxic preparations, until a point is reached where the insecticides threaten to become more dangerous in the long run to the human species than to the insects for which they are intended. The need to rescue a crop from agricultural mismanagement gains priority over the health and well-being of the consumer. The use of drugs to fatten and accelerate the growth of domestic animals is playing havoc with the physiology of our livestock. The damage these drugs inflict on poultry and cattle necessitates the use of additional drugs, which, in turn, contaminate man's food and reduce the value of these agents in combating disease. It would seem to be a form of ecological retribution that the very forces man has summoned against the living world around him are being redirected by a remorseless logic against the human organism itself.

CHEMICALS IN FOOD PROCESSING

THE SAME OVERCOMMITMENT to potentially risky methods is found in other phases of food production. Complex problems of storage, cleansing, handling, refining,
cooking, mixing, heating, and packaging are often
solved by the use of chemical additives. A half century
ago the yellowish tint in freshly milled flour was removed
slowly by aging; today it is removed rapidly by oxidizing
agents. The miller no longer has to store flour and wait
for it to mature. Emulsifiers are employed, partly to "improve" the texture of a product, partly to speed up processing. Their "functional advantages" in ice cream, for example, are that the "mix can be whipped faster, the
product from the freezer is dryer, and the mix has less
tendency to 'churn' in the freezer." Chemical antioxidants
are used to help prevent oils and fats from becoming
rancid, a problem that becomes especially pronounced
when natural antioxidants are removed during large-
scale processing. Chemical preservatives are added to
food to permit longer storage in wholesale depots and to
extend the "shelf life" of a product in retail outlets. In
time chemicals are turned from mere adjuncts of food
production into "technological necessities." Their use may
result in new machines and facilities, the abandonment
of old processing methods, and a broad reorientation of
technology to meet the new chemical requirements.

The fact that a chemical is technologically useful
does not mean that it is biologically desirable. The two
phrases are occasionally used interchangeably, as though
they were synonymous. Some of the chemicals most
widely used in the production of food have been found to
be harmful to animals in laboratory tests. Nitrogen tri-

chloride, or agene, was employed for decades as a bleaching and maturing agent in flour before it was discovered, in 1946, that the compound produces "running fits," or hysteria, in dogs. The use of agene in the bread industry has since been discontinued. Although there is no evidence that agenized flour causes nerve disorders in man, no one can say with certainty that cereal products treated with agene are completely harmless to consumers, especially if eaten day after day for twenty years or more. The toxicant in agenized flour "produces nervous disturbances in monkeys, but not epilepsy in man," observed the late Anton Carlson, one of the most distinguished physiologists of his day. "That is not sufficient for me, because there are many other types of nervous disturbances . . . that may be aggravated or introduced by this chemical."

Another group of chemicals, notably certain types of polyoxyethylene derivatives, were widely used in the United States as emulsifiers before they were banned as potential hazards to consumers. Former F.D.A. Commissioner Charles W. Crawford is reported to have described the agents as "good paint removers." According to data furnished to the Delaney Committee, rats that had been fed two commercial preparations of polyoxyethylene-derived emulsifiers showed blood in their feces and developed a variety of kidney, abdominal, cardiac, and liver abnormalities. These preparations were used primarily as bread softeners but also found their way into other foods. The polyoxyethylene derivatives constitute a highly suspect family of emulsifying agents, yet some of them are still added to cake mixes, cake icing, frozen desserts, ice cream, candies, dill pickles, fruit and vegetable coatings, vitamin preparations, and many food-packaging materials.*

* Several experiments indicate that an intake of large amounts of polyoxyethylene (8) stearate produces gall stones and bladder

Similar examples can be culled from other groups of chemical aids. In general, the toxic effects of many commonly used compounds are difficult to determine, but individually and in groups they have aroused suspicion and concern. "The fortification of oils and fats against oxidation and rancidity is another field in which there are serious questions of possible toxicity," warns F. J. Schlink, technical director of Consumers' Research and editor of *Consumer Bulletin*. "The natural antioxidants which delay rancidity are lost during the factory processing of refined oils and fats; then the attempt is made to restore the antioxidation qualities by addition of fat-stabilizing substances. Most of the materials that have antioxidation properties are known to be toxic to some degree."

The term "technological aid" has been used loosely to include food additives that could be dispensed with entirely if a manufacturer improved his processing methods and the quality of his product. The question of whether a chemical, instead of being legitimately employed to furnish distant consumers with a perishable product, was being used rather as a device for masking inferior ingredients and unsanitary methods arose in sharp form early in the century, when sodium benzoate was employed extensively as a preservative in catsup. Harvey Wiley, the first administrator of the federal food and drug law, regarded sodium benzoate as a hazard to consumers. Supported by data from feeding experiments performed with human beings, Wiley claimed that the

---

tumors in rats. At least two commercial preparations of polyoxyethylene derivatives are reported to be co-carcinogens; they promote the development of skin cancer in mice when used in conjunction with certain carcinogenic agents. For a number of years all three of these polyoxyethylene compounds were used as food additives in the United States. By the early 1950's, polyoxyethylene derivatives had also migrated to England, where they were used on a limited scale as bread softeners.

preservative causes injury to the digestive system. He was convinced that catsup need not deteriorate readily if clean facilities and proper ingredients are used in preparing it. Challenged on this point by Charles F. Loudon, a canner in Terre Haute, Indiana, Wiley appointed a bacteriologist, Arvill W. Bitting, to work at the Loudon factory and prepare a formula for a stable catsup preparation without artificial preservatives. Bitting was successful. Moreover, after inspecting numerous canning factories and examining many brands of catsup, Bitting concluded that manufacturers who needed sodium benzoate often used inferior products and were careless about sanitation.

"The whole spirit and tradition of the pure-food law is against the use of preservatives and substitutes," declared Mrs. Harvey Wiley more than forty years after the Loudon episode. "The intent of the law is to encourage the manufacture of high-grade ingredients, not to try to hide inferiority and cheapness by the use of chemicals and preservatives." If this is so, the spirit of the law has been ignored for decades. The most up-to-date surveys of chemical additives in foods show that preservatives are added to cheese, margarine, cereal products, jams, jelly, and many other processed foods. Uncooked poultry is dipped in solutions of antibiotics.* Aside from the damage to public health that may arise from the use of questionable chemicals as preservatives, the longer "shelf life" acquired by some of these foods may cause a loss of valuable nutrients.

Many chemical additives in foods perform no technological or nutritional function whatever. They cannot

---

* Notably the tetracyclines. Despite strong pressure from the food industry, the British Food Standards Committee has refused to recommend the use of tetracyclines as preservatives for poultry and fish.

be regarded as materially useful by any stretch of the imagination. These chemicals enhance the color of a food or make certain products feel soft and newly prepared; in some instances they have been used to replace costly but valuable nutrients with inferior ones. In the least objectionable cases, an additive will deceive the consumer without impairing his health. The application of an innocuous vegetable dye to some foods often leads the consumer to believe that he is acquiring a better, more wholesome, or tastier product than is actually the case. In the most objectionable cases, a chemical is toxic to a greater or lesser degree. This type of additive not only serves to change the appearance or conceal the nutritive deficiency of a food; it exposes the consumer to a certain amount of damage.

Nitrates and nitrites, for example, are used to impart a pink color to certain brands of processed meat. Ostensibly, this is their sole function. The addition of these chemicals to meat, especially frankfurters and hamburger meat, would be objectionable if only because of the deception which makes it difficult for the housewife to distinguish between high-quality and low-quality products. But this is not the only deception perpetrated on the consumer. Used together with salt, nitrite compounds definitely extend the "shelf life" of processed meat products.

When nitrites are ingested, they react with hemoglobin in the blood to form methemoglobin, and, like carbon monoxide, reduce the hemoglobin's capacity to carry oxygen. An individual who consumes three to four ounces of processed meat containing 200 parts per million of sodium nitrite (a permissible residue) ingests enough of the compound to convert from 1.4 to 5.7 per cent of his hemoglobin to methemoglobin. Ordinarily, this percentage is insignificant. But if the same individual is a heavy smoker and lives in an air-polluted community, the cumulative loss in oxygen-carrying capacity produced by the nitrites in the food and by the carbon monoxide in tobacco smoke and motorcar exhaust can no longer be dismissed as trivial. Sodium nitrite is highly toxic in relatively small amounts. About four grams of the compound constitutes a lethal dose for adults. Although Lehman regards 200 parts per million of sodium nitrite as a safe residue, he notes that "only a small margin of safety exists between the amount of nitrite that is safe and that which may be dangerous. The margin of safety is even more reduced when the smaller blood volume and the corresponding smaller quantity of hemoglobin in children is taken into account. This has been emphasized in the recent cases of nitrite poisoning in children who consumed weiners and bologna containing nitrite greatly in excess of the 200 ppm permitted by Federal regulations. The application of nitrite to other foods is not to be encouraged."

Emulsifiers have been used in bread not only as softening agents, which can give stale bread the texture of newly baked bread, but as substitutes for nourishing ingredients. "The record of the bread-standards hearings contain evidence of distribution among bakers of advertising material advocating the replacement of fats, oils, eggs, and milk by emulsifiers," George L. Prichard, of the Department of Agriculture, told the Delaney Committee. "The use of such products as components of food may work to the disadvantage of our farm economy by displacing farm products normally used. The record indicates that natural food constituents, such as fats and oils, probably will be reduced in many commercial bakery products if bakers are allowed to employ these emulsifiers."

This substitution affects more than the farm economy, however; it also works to the disadvantage of the consumer. To illustrate this, the Delaney Committee report compared the ingredients in two cake batters prepared by the same company eleven years apart; during the interval emulsifiers were added to the product. The first batter, made in 1939, did not contain synthetic emulsifiers; the second, prepared in 1949, did. "On a percentage basis, the cake batter in 1939 contained 13 per cent eggs, and 8.6 per cent shortening. In 1949, the cake batter contained 6.3 per cent eggs, and 4.8 per cent shortening, with somewhat less than 0.3 per cent of synthetic emulsifier." The report noted that a "synthetic yellow dye could be added to provide the color formerly obtainable through the use of eggs. The utilization of synthetic yellow dye in commercial cake was practiced before the war. There are indications that the use of artificial coloring matter is increased when quantities of whole eggs or egg yolks are reduced in commercial cake formulas."

To heighten the insult, among the most commonly used emulsifiers in 1949 were the polyoxyethylene monostearates. The yellow dye referred to in the Delaney Committee report was probably FDC Yellow No. 3 (Yellow AB), which, until fairly recently, was added to many yellow cake mixes. As we shall see in the following chapter, the dye often contained impurities of a potent carcinogen and its use in foods was forbidden in 1959. For a number of years, however, both the emulsifier and the dye undoubtedly appeared in many brands of cake and reached large numbers of unsuspecting consumers.

Problems of this kind are not likely to disappear unless there is a basic change in the viewpoint of the F.D.A. "Inherited from the Wiley era is a too common misconception that all 'chemicals' are harmful, and the related idea that any amount of a 'poison' is harmful," the F.D.A. observes in a brochure on food additives. "The fact is, of course, that chemical additives, or *food additives* as they are now being called, have brought about great improvements in the American food supply. Additives like potassium iodide in salt and vitamins in enriched food products are making an important contribution to the health of our people, and yet it is a fact that both iodine and some of the vitamins would be harmful if consumed in excessive amounts. Many similar examples could be given to refute these common misconceptions."

This argument is grossly misleading. Iodine and vitamins are indispensable to human life, but coal-tar dyes and benzoic acid, for example, are not. If we adhered to a well-balanced diet of properly prepared natural foods, iodine and vitamins would never enter the body in toxic amounts. Coal-tar dyes, on the other hand, are suspected of being harmful to man in nearly any amount if consumed repeatedly, and the kindest statement that can be made for the presence of benzoic acid in food is that the compound is "safe under the conditions of its intended use."

The formula "safe under the conditions of its intended use" exposes the consumer to serious risks when it opens the door to the use of food additives whose biochemical activity is not understood. Many unexpected problems may arise when such additives appear in food. A particular additive may seem to be relatively harmless to the organs of the body, but it may be carcinogenic on the cellular level of life. Another additive may produce insignificant or controllable effects when studied in isolation; brought into combination with various chemicals in food, however, it may give rise to toxic compounds. The body, in turn, may make a toxic additive more poisonous in the course of changing it during metabolism. "At one time it was generally believed that whenever a toxic substance was absorbed the body was capable of calling upon special mechanisms for detoxifying the toxicant," Lehman observes. "It was believed also that the metabolic pathway that the toxicant followed always proceeded in the direction of the formation of a less toxic compound. Later work on the metabolism of drugs and toxic substances showed that special mechanisms did not exist, but that the toxicant was subject to the same metabolic influences as those which normally operate in the body. The assumption that the metabolic product was less poisonous than the parent substance from which it was derived is also unwarranted simply because in many instances the toxicity of either the original substance and its conversion product is unknown. In other instances the metabolic product is even more poisonous than its parent. The conversion product, heptachlorepoxide, which is two or three times more poisonous than the parent substance, heptachlor [a widely used insecticide], may be cited as an example of this."

Finally, food additives may cause allergic reactions that are likely to go unnoticed for many years. The reactions need not be severe to be harmful. Otto Saphir and his colleagues at the Michael Reese Hospital in Chicago have recently suggested that the development of arteriosclerosis may be promoted by the sensitivity of the body to allergenic compounds, notably certain antibiotics. By using sulfa drugs to produce allergies in forty-two rabbits, the researchers were able in eight months to cause degenerative changes in the arteries of thirty-one of the animals. These changes closely resembled arteriosclerosis in man. According to a press account of Saphir's report, the rabbits' reactions "were not apparent on the surface." It would be very imprudent to assume that such effects are produced only by chemicals that cause severe or noticeable allergies. If the data of Saphir and his colleagues are applicable to man, additives with even minor allergenic properties cannot be dismissed as harmless.

Today more than 3,000 chemicals are used in the production and distribution of commercially prepared food. At least 1,288 are purposely added as preservatives, buffers, emulsifiers, neutralizing agents, sequestrants, stabilizers, anticaking agents, flavoring agents, and coloring agents, while from 25 to 30 consist of nutritional supplements, such as potassium iodide and vitamins. The remaining chemicals are "indirect additives"—substances, such as detergents and germicides, that get into food by way of packaging materials and processing equipment. Many chemical additives are natural ingredients, but a large number are not. The artificial substances that appear in food range from simple inorganic chemicals to exotic compounds whose biochemical activity is still largely unknown.

At a time when almost every processed food contains chemical additives or residues, the "misconceptions" of the "Wiley era" must seem like bold anticipations. Sixty years ago the number of chemicals added to food was small. Public concern was aroused primarily by the gross adulteration of food and by the unsanitary practices followed in mills and slaughterhouses. These problems are still with us; as recently as 1958, over 5,000 tons of food was seized by the F.D.A. because of filth and decomposition. But the problem of chemicals in food has reached proportions that would have appalled Wiley, and the incidence of diseases, such as cancer, that can be produced by chemicals in man's environment has increased to an alarming extent. We sense that our food technology has taken a wrong turn. Having achieved the abundance of nutriment it once promised, it threatens to become another factor imperiling man's health and well-being.

CHAPTER FIVE

Environment and Cancer

THE IMPORTANCE OF ENVIRONMENT

ONE OF THE most challenging problems in public health involves the influence of man's environment on the incidence of cancer. Differences of opinion concerning the extent of this influence are likely to have important practical consequences. If a specialist believes that cancer is caused primarily by genetic factors or by the aging process, his hopes for controlling the disease will focus on advances in surgery, radiology, and chemical therapy. He will tend to regard the occurrence of the disease as inevitable. On the other hand, if he strongly suspects that environmental factors play a major role, he is likely to attach a great deal of importance to cancer prevention. He will regard environmental change as a serious problem requiring careful investigation. Nothing can be done to arrest the aging process or alter the individual's genetic endowment, but almost any environmental factor that influences the incidence of cancer is subject to some degree of social or individual control. The more effectively control is exercised, the lower the incidence of cancer is likely to be.

To what extent, then, are the two points of view supported by evidence and scientific authority?

Fortunately, it has never been established that cancer results from the aging process. At most it has been shown that the highest incidence of certain types of cancer occurs in the later years of life—a fact that can be explained by the longer exposure of older people to cancer-causing substances. "The senescence theory does no more than paraphrase a fact," notes Sigismund Peller; "it fails to indicate how and where the changes are initiated which end in cancer." The theory that cancer is inheritable rests on more impressive evidence and, for a time, occupied a commanding position in cancer research. It had its greatest following in the 1920's, when Maud Slye managed to produce highly inbred strains of mice in which nearly every specimen acquired a cancer. Even the type of cancer and the age at which it appeared could be predicted with reasonable and often astonishing accuracy. Miss Slye advanced the view that cancer is due to a single genetic factor that determines nearly every aspect of the disease—the type of cancer, the site on which it arises, and the age at which it appears. Whether an individual acquired a cancer or not seemed to depend almost entirely upon his genetic endowment.

But the world is not a genetics laboratory in which individuals are mated to prove a point about hereditary cancer. Fortunately, examples of hereditary cancer in man are rare. After further research, it became evident that seemingly hereditary cancers in certain highly inbred strains of mice depended upon a complex of non-genetic factors. In experiments with one of the most "inheritable" forms of the disease—breast cancer in the mouse—Bittner demonstrated "that the kind of milk given to a litter accounts for more than all hereditary factors together. Whether a high or low probability of spontaneous breast cancer may be expected depends primarily upon the milk (mother versus foster mother taken from a different strain) which the new born mouse of a genetically pure strain sucks in the first twenty-four hours after birth." Bittner's "milk factor" is now believed to be a virus. Clarence Little found that the susceptibility of inbred mice to certain tumor grafts could not be explained without taking at least fourteen different genes into account, and even then many problems arose when the tumors were transplanted. Although a predisposition to cancer may be inherited, it is difficult to believe that an individual is foredoomed to acquire the disease by a genetic factor. "On the contrary," observes Charles Oberling, director of the Institute of Cancer Research in Paris, "cancerous heredity is discovered to be a mosaic of factors that intervene in the most varied domains of the anatomic, physiological, and immunological constitution and cooperate in preparing a soil that is favorable for the emergence of a malignant neoplasm."

It is tempting to add that if the "soil" is prepared by heredity, the "seed" is planted by the environment. A predisposition to cancer is not an absolute that is either present or absent; it is a matter of degree, varying from person to person. It is likely to manifest itself in malignant tumors to the extent that individuals are exposed to carcinogens. The greater the exposure, the higher the incidence of cancer. In fact, cases are known in which the activity of a particular carcinogen largely determines the rate of death from cancer. For example, Peller found that cancer accounted for 51 per cent of the deaths among the radium miners of Joachimsthal in Czechoslovakia. More than half the miners in this community were confronted with the prospect of dying of cancer, an appallingly high percentage. As cancer "normally" accounts for 20 per cent of the adult mortality rate, Peller reasons, approximately 39 per cent of those who might never have succumbed to the disease died of it. In these circumstances, variations in individual predispositions to cancer are so much overshadowed by the potency of a carcinogen (radon) that the "seed" can germinate virtually without any "soil" prepared by hereditary or constitutional factors.

Indeed, one may well ask: What is a "normal" cancer death rate? Is the toll predetermined by genetic factors or will rates vary markedly in different environments? The most reliable evidence at hand suggests that the incidence of cancer and the number of lives claimed by the disease vary appreciably from one kind of environment to another, even within the same general region. An extensive survey of cancer illness in Iowa during 1951, for example, showed that the incidence of the disease was proportionately almost 40 per cent higher in urban areas of the state than in rural areas. Although large differences could be expected in the incidence of lung cancer, it is noteworthy that a higher rate was reported among city dwellers for all forms of cancer. Urban women had a 25 per cent higher incidence of breast cancer and a 50 per cent higher incidence of genital cancer. Surprisingly, urban men had a much higher incidence of skin cancer (45 per cent), despite the fact that people in rural areas are exposed to greater amounts of sunlight, a natural carcinogen. These variations could not be accounted for by any differences in the quality of medical services or in access to hospitals and doctors. "Rural areas in Iowa appear to have access to the same degree and quality of medical care that urban areas have. Also, the cancer incidence rates for rural areas in metropolitan counties were no higher than for rural areas in remote non-metropolitan counties."

In addition, the incidence of cancer is higher among certain income groups and occupations. The disease occurs most frequently in the poorest strata of the metropolis. Harold F. Dorn and Sidney J. Cutler found that among "white females the incidence of cancer was 14 per cent above average in the lowest income class, but occurred with about equal frequency in the four other income classes. . . . The most consistent relationship is the observation of relatively high incidence among members of the lower income classes." Although a few forms of cancer show a mild preference for the rich, most types appear with the greatest frequency among the urban poor. Workers who are exposed to industrial carcinogens have a higher incidence of cancer than clerks, and those in nearly all major urban occupations have relatively more cases of the disease than do farmers.

Viewed in this perspective, cancer seems to have certain features in common with tuberculosis. Although the two diseases are fundamentally different in many respects, it is noteworthy that the incidence of both cancer and tuberculosis increases with urbanization. Nor can we overlook the fact that cancer, like tuberculosis, claims the largest number of its victims from among the urban poor. The organs in which the diseases take root "are not only determined by the properties of the particular pathogenic [disease-causing] agent involved, but also by the type or route of contact with it," observes W. C. Hueper. "The conditions of exposure which decide the development of tuberculosis of the lungs and of the intestine—inhalation and ingestion, respectively—are fundamentally no different from those which are responsible for the development of cancers of the skin, bones, lungs, etc., after exposure to radioactive material by skin contact, inhalation, ingestion, or parenteral introduction."

Tuberculosis became pandemic only after man's environment underwent a radical change. Although rural workers were familiar with hunger before the Industrial Revolution, they seldom contracted tuberculosis in large numbers, partly because they lived in open surroundings and engaged in healthful work. The disease, we may recall, turned into the "white plague" when men were crowded into large cities and overworked in dismal factories. It spread among them rapidly even though, in certain cases, they were getting more to eat. Tuberculosis-promoting factors overshadowed advances that might well have prevented a high incidence of infection. Today we know that control of the disease is achieved primarily through social advances, better sanitation, and improvement of the standard of living.

The same attention to all the aspects of our environment may be required to control cancer. There is good reason to believe that nearly everything that seriously disturbs the proper functioning of the human organism, particularly many of the toxicants produced by the present-day industrial revolution, contributes to the incidence of the disease. We shall find that cancer is promoted by emotional stress, poor diet, and a large variety of environmental pollutants. While the disease remains a "riddle," to borrow Oberling's word, it threatens to become the major cause of death in the United States and western Europe. In 1945 one out of every eight Americans was expected to die of the disease; today the figure is one out of six. Twenty-five per cent of the population now living in the United States will eventually acquire cancer, and approximately 450,000 new cases of the disease are discovered annually. Sweeping environmental changes in the nineteenth century produced the "white plague"— pandemic tuberculosis; changes in the present century seem to have spawned a "gray plague"—pandemic cancer.

The complexity of the disease should not be underestimated. It is highly improbable that any cancers arise "spontaneously," that is, in the absence of a carcinogen. Whether a carcinogen initiates a series of changes in a cell or is continuously involved in them, the biochemical reactions that lead to malignant tumors often occur in stages, many of which are manifested by abnormalities in pre-cancerous tissue. Whether it is in the stomach, the uterus, or the prostate gland, "cancer rarely appears as a bolt from the blue," Oberling observes. "Almost always it is preceded by nutritional disturbances in the epithelium that masquerade under various names but that are, after all, merely the expression of an abnormal reactivity to certain influences."

Many cancer specialists believe that once a cell is altered by a carcinogen, the change is irreversible; the cell acquires an "imprint" and transmits it to all its descendants. Whether or not a cancer develops depends upon many factors, such as the potency of the carcinogen, the extent of exposure to other chemical and physical agents, and the individual's constitution. Malignant cells may become detached from a localized cancer and enter the blood stream without producing new tumors. Apparently, certain resistance mechanisms must be overcome before malignant cells can take root elsewhere in the body and produce invasive, secondary cancers.

A cancer can be induced by a single chemical agent or by several, by small, irregular doses of the carcinogen or by a few large ones. The disease may not manifest itself for many years, even decades. A carcinogen may reach man by way of the air he breathes, the fluids he drinks, and the food he eats. It may harm a specific part of the body or the organism as a whole. Any powerful agent or stimulus that alters the normal functioning of human metabolism over a long period of time is potentially carcinogenic. Let us concede that the word "normal" has yet to be defined and that each individual has different biological needs. But let us also acknowledge that the incidence of cancer can be increased enormously by reckless changes in man's environment, that millions of lives are placed in jeopardy by thoughtless alterations in man's manner of life, diet, and physical surroundings.

THE GENERAL ENVIRONMENT

WHAT ARE SOME of the general, or nonspecific, factors that influence the onset and progress of cancer? If this question is often difficult to answer, the reason is not that these factors are too few; on the contrary, there are too many of them, and the problem is to decide which ones are the most important. There is evidence that both the occurrence of a cancer and its course are influenced by the subject's emotional make-up, his diet, and his occupation. The adequate treatment of a cancer, in turn, requires knowledge not only of surgery, radiation, and chemical therapeutics but also of the patient's character and environment. Although the course of many cancers is generally predictable, individual responses to treatment vary so widely that a specific cancer that usually causes death within a few months can, in some cases, be controlled for several years.

Emotional stress is an important element in the

progress of certain cancers. At the annual meeting of the American Cancer Society in 1959, several cancer specialists focused attention on the role that anxiety seems to play in the onset and course of malignant tumors. Drawing upon his experiences as a radiologist, Eugene P. Pendergrass, the outgoing president of the society, observed that even if psychological factors do not determine the eventual outcome of cancer, they seem to influence the development of the disease. "I personally have observed cancer patients who had undergone successful treatment and were living well for years. Then an emotional stress such as a death of a son in World War II, the infidelity of a daughter-in-law, or the burden of long unemployment seems to have been a precipitating factor in the reactivation of their disease which resulted in death." A similar viewpoint was expressed by John B. Graham, of the Roswell Park Memorial Institute in Buffalo. "The adversities and despairs that these people [cancer victims] are subject to, and their responses to them, are indeed factors in the development of cancer and the effectiveness of treatment." At a press conference, Graham added: "It has seemed to us in some cases that despair precedes cancer. I would not say it is a cause, but it may be a factor which decides when cancer will develop."

In view of what we know of Selye's work on stress and the adrenal corticoids, these conclusions should not be surprising. Cortisone is used effectively to delay death in cases of such hopeless cancers as acute leukemia. The temporary remissions achieved by this hormone are often striking. After being treated with cortisone, a victim of acute leukemia often seems to be on the point of complete recovery, although in time the cancer invariably overcomes the effects achieved by the hormone. There are reasons for suspecting that, just as cortisone inhibits the growth of certain cancers, other adrenal hormones sustain and even propagate cancers of the breast and prostate gland. By removing the adrenal glands of patients suffering from these tumors, physicians often gain control of the disease for long periods of time. New methods are replacing adrenal surgery, but the inhibition of the production of corticoids is a basic technique in managing both types of cancer. According to Selye, the value of adrenal surgery in certain cases of cancer "would suggest that there are adrenal factors which stimulate cancer formation."

It is tempting to speculate whether emotional stress, by influencing the output of the adrenal glands, contributes significantly to the rising incidence of cancer. The adrenal cortex normally secretes male sex hormones (androgens) and perhaps female sex hormones (estrogens). The corticoids are also directly involved in the secretion of hormones by the male and female sex glands. Many experiments have shown that injections of estrogens induce mammary cancer in cancer-prone mice, and intensive use of estrogen to control cancer of the prostate gland in men has been followed, in some cases, by breast cancer. "There can be little doubt that endocrine imbalance is the basis for chronic cystic mastitis, or *maladie de Reclus,* which is characterized by fibrous nodules that are sometimes interspersed with cysts, and it has been shown by Warren and by Foote and Stewart that cancer is five times as common in breasts affected by this condition as it is in normal ones."

Oberling's opinion, advanced in 1952, received strong support several years later from the results of autopsies performed on 207 women with cancers of the breast. The investigators found evidence of marked endocrine imbalances and particularly of prolonged estrogenic stimulation of tissues in the breasts. Like the corticoids, the estrogens are steroids, and there is a close resemblance between the chemical structure of the steroid hormones and that of certain carcinogens. Some of these carcinogens, in turn, have a mild estrogenic activity; that is, they produce, on a smaller scale, effects similar to those produced by estrogens and corticoids. There is a possibility either that excessive secretions of the steroids turn precancerous cells into cancerous ones or that the hormones are actually degraded into carcinogens. At any rate, the apparent relationships between stress and cancer and between the steroids and carcinogens can hardly be ignored.

"There is solid evidence that the course of disease, in general, is affected by emotional stress," Pendergrass observes. "A growing list of authorities have lent support to this field of investigation. Foremost among these is Dr. Hans Selye who devoted much of his life to the subject. In order to learn about such stresses, one must explore beyond the usual limits of a clinical history. This takes time. Busy doctors may be unable to give the time to secure a good history concerned with environmental, constitutional and other factors; a history of emotional stress, or just the opposite; a climate of happiness and security. Could this not be an area for another discipline in medicine, [for] a social scientist for instance; or maybe this is a field where the social worker should expand his or her activities. I believe that research in this area will, almost certainly, lead into investigations of factors that are susceptible to control hormonal systems and other general metabolic influences. Thus, we as doctors may begin to emphasize *treatment of the patient as a whole*, as well as the disease from which the patient is suffering. We may learn how to influence the general body systems and through them modify the neoplasm which resides within the body."

Cancer does not always grind inexorably to its logical end. At least 150 spontaneous remissions of cancer in man have been carefully authenticated by reputable scientists. A number of these tumors had already metastasized widely and were regarded as incurable. As Oberling observes: ". . . it is difficult to estimate the frequency of spontaneous cure because cancer is generally not recognized until it has reached an advanced stage. It is entirely possible that many malignant growths disappear in their initial stages, leaving no trace behind. This, of course, is the purest speculation."

But Oberling's speculation is not reckless. Research has clearly demonstrated that organisms possess mechanisms for resisting cancer. According to a report by the Sloan-Kettering Institute for Cancer Research, defense mechanisms have been observed in mice receiving transplants of a highly malignant cancer which usually kills 95 per cent of its victims in three weeks. "If these animals were given a small dose of material extracted from yeast cells called zymosan, they defended themselves vigorously against the cancer. Instead of killing the mice, the cancers were gradually dissolved until they disappeared entirely. The animals were then completely cured. No cancer has ever returned, and strong immunity to a second implantation has been demonstrated as long as 11 months after the first growth was initiated. Remarkably, these cancer cells grown in tissue culture are not disturbed at all when put in direct contact with zymosan. This indicates that zymosan does not inhibit the cancer directly but acts in some way in mice to enhance their natural defenses, tipping the scales in favor of the endangered host and against the cancer." The yeast extract, unfortunately, "is too toxic in man for clinical use."

This line of research is important because high resistance depends not only on hereditary factors but also on good nutrition, a sound state of mind, and balance in work and play. It is fairly well established that the high incidence of liver cancers in depressed areas of the world is due in large part to dietary deficiencies of protein and possibly the B vitamins. Rats nourished on similarly deficient diets have a high incidence of the disease, although it is rare in animals that receive the same food supplemented with wheat, yeast, or powdered liver. Dietary factors may also contribute to the relatively high incidence of chorioepithelioma (a cancer of the uterus) in the Far East. In general, however, experimental data are inconclusive for other forms of cancer because the relationship between animal tumors and nutrition varies with the strain and species used. "It does appear that maintenance of body weight at a minimum compatible with good health may prevent or delay the development of cancer in many individuals," observes Helen N. Lovell in a review of the available evidence. "A diet adequate in all nutrients seems to be most desirable. Many believe the oral and pharyngeal symptoms of chronic riboflavin and nicotinic acid deficiency are precancerous factors."

Despite the influence of all the factors we have been discussing, many well-nourished and serene individuals perish from virulent cancers fairly early in life. Why? What are some of the factors that might produce malignant tumors in persons whose diet, habits, and outlook are sound? These questions introduce a formidable problem. Man is exposed to a large number of cancer-causing agents; some of them are natural in origin and virtually impossible to avoid, but a substantial number of them are man-made. A few of these artificial agents are useful in medicine, but the majority can be either completely dispensed with or at least used in such a way that they do not affect the general public. The presence of these agents in the human environment has aroused a great deal of concern, and their removal requires vigorous social action.

THE CHEMICAL CARCINOGENS

MAN IS CAPABLE of producing at least two types of agents that have cancer-causing properties. One of them, ionizing radiation, will be discussed at some length in the following chapter. Our principal concern here will be with the chemical carcinogens, ranging from confirmed cancer-causing substances to those that are highly suspect.

The suspicion that chemicals in man's environment can cause cancer first arose nearly two centuries ago, when Sir Percival Pott, a London surgeon, identified "chimney sweep's disease" as cancer of the scrotum. Pott unerringly pointed to soot, the tarry material formed by the combustion of solid fuels, as the cause of this malignant tumor. In the eighteenth century the job of cleaning chimneys was given to boys who were small enough to negotiate the elaborate flues in the London homes of that period. As the boys worked, their trousers rubbed soot into the sweat glands of the scrotum. In later life, perhaps ten or fifteen years after this kind of work had been abandoned, the scrotum would begin to ulcerate and then develop a cancer which invariably claimed the life of its victim. In 1914 two Japanese investigators, K. Yamagiwa and K. Itchikawa, succeeded in developing skin cancer in 41 of 178 rabbits who had received applications of tar to the internal surface of the ear. Three years later H. Tsutsui was able to similarly induce tar cancer in mice.

The success of these Japanese investigators met with warm professional appreciation—and for good reason. Their work opened a new era in cancer research—the study of chemical carcinogens—and with it there arose a host of disconcerting problems concerning the behavior of these agents in men and animals.

Yamagiwa and Itchikawa would not have been able to produce tar cancer of the skin if they had used guinea pigs instead of rabbits. Although tar induces cancer in man, it does not produce the disease in the guinea pig, an animal commonly used in experimental work. In all probability, the Japanese investigators would also have been unsuccessful if they had used rats. Despite repeated attempts from 1914 on, cancer of the skin could not be produced in this animal through applications of tar until 1935. They might also have failed with dogs, whose response to tar is "sporadic and inconstant," in Oberling's words. In short, evidence that tar is carcinogenic in animals was acquired partly through luck and partly through patience. Yamagiwa and Itchikawa had the good fortune to select an animal that is more susceptible to tar cancer than other experimental subjects, but they had to persevere through at least 150 applications of the carcinogen before malignant tumors were induced.

Their experiment was not the first attempt to induce cancer in animals by means of tar. Similar efforts were made in 1888, 1890, and 1894, and again as late as 1913, by Haga, another Japanese investigator. All the attempts failed. The experiments in the last two decades of the nineteenth century were performed mostly on dogs and rats. Haga even turned to the rabbit as a subject, but he failed to keep at the tar applications long enough. The medical pundits of the day thereupon concluded that chemical carcinogenesis did not exist. "For decades these few negative [experimental] results weighed more heavily than numerous observations to the contrary in chimney sweeps, tar, paraffin and dye workers, and mule spinners," Peller observes. ". . . only after positive experimental results on animals had been published, did cancerologists change their opinions. It was formerly considered scientifically sound to deny the relationship; now it became sound to accept it. If Yamagiwa and Itchikawa (1914) and Tsutsui (1917) had chosen the rat for their experiments, instead of rabbits and mice, then the tar genesis of certain skin epitheliomas in man and the theory of irritation in cancer would have been 'expertly' denied for another 17 to 20 years, and the whole development of chemistry of cancerogens would have been retarded."

The same story can be told about beta-naphthalamine, a compound used in the preparation of a number of coal-tar dyes. Beta-naphthalamine, which induces cancer of the bladder, is one of the most potent carcinogenic substances in man's environment; it has claimed hundreds of lives among workers in the synthetic-dye industry. Attempts were made as early as 1906 to induce cancer in rabbits by means of synthetic dyes, including beta-naphthalamine, but the experimenter, B. Fischer, did not persist long enough in his efforts. After producing cancerlike cells that regressed spontaneously when injections of the carcinogens were stopped, Fischer concluded that the dyes did not induce occupational cancers. This conclusion was generally accepted by the medical profession. Not until the late 1920's were cancers produced experimentally by beta-naphthalamine, but even then rabbits proved to be poor subjects and rats and mice were found to be resistant to the compound. In 1938, more than thirty years after Fischer's work, Hueper and his coworkers discovered that the only animal that readily contracted cancer of the bladder from beta-naphthalamine was the dog.

The reason for inflicting these details on the reader should be fairly obvious. Cancers in animals "cannot provide irrefutable proof of the safety or carcinogenicity of a substance for the human species," observes a report by the Food Protection Committee of the National Academy of Sciences. The committee adds that "it is perhaps reassuring that the known carcinogenic responses of humans to certain chemicals are similar in many ways to those seen in experimental animals"—but the qualifying words "perhaps," "certain," and "in many ways" carry a heavy burden. Actually, some carcinogens are handled quite differently in man from the way they are handled in common experimental animals. Beta-naphthalamine, for example, is not carcinogenic as such. In the human body, however, it is metabolized into the carcinogen 2-amino-1-naphthol, whereas resistant animals either fail to produce this metabolic compound or create it in very small amounts.

Many subtle physiological differences between animal species—indeed, between individuals in the same species—are likely to affect the potency of a chemical carcinogen. "The only universal carcinogen is apparently ionizing radiation," Hueper notes. Whether or not a cancer is produced by an environmental carcinogen depends on the organ with which it comes in contact, on the solubility of the carcinogen in the body's fluids and therefore "on the speed of removal from the site of primary contact of a carcinogen, upon the metabolism of the carcinogen, on its route of excretion and on the tissue or organ of retention or deposition of a carcinogen. The target organ may vary in different species." Hueper concludes that the ability of a carcinogen to affect different species and organs in different ways seems to depend on the distinctive metabolic processes of the animals involved.

These factors apparently account for the fact that several types of cancer that are common in man are difficult to produce in animals. For example, until very recently the most common form of stomach cancer in humans (adenocarcinoma) could not be produced in rabbits, mice, rats, and dogs by feeding them various carcinogens. On the other hand, adenocarcinomas of the small intestine, while rare in man, are fairly easy to produce in animals. The lung tumors produced in mice do not resemble the lung tumors in humans that have aroused so much professional and public concern. Many cancer specialists even disagree on whether these tumors in mice are malignant or benign. Spontaneous regressions of cancer in mice, animals widely used in cancer research, are not uncommon, but the regression of diagnosed cancers is very rare in man.

When the researcher finds that a particular compound does not induce cancer in rats, mice, or dogs, he can only hope that it will not cause the disease in man. He can never be certain of this unless carefully controlled experiments on a large number of human volunteers are continued for decades without causing a cancer that is clearly attributable to the particular chemical. Experiments with animals are likely to be more painstaking if the compound being tested is chemically related to a number of known carcinogens. But there are no clear-cut groups of carcinogenic substances. Some known carcinogens are highly complex hydrocarbons; others, such as chromium, nickel, and arsenic, usually reach man as simple inorganic compounds. Often the most trivial chemical change can transform an apparently non-carcinogenic substance into a potent carcinogen. A mere shift of the NH_2 group in alpha-naphthalamine, a non-carcinogenic compound, from one position to another in the molecular ring of the chemical produces the carcinogen beta-naphthalamine.

Many carcinogens have been able to enter man's environment because of the relative crudeness of experimental techniques. Even today, despite advances in testing methods, carcinogenic properties are being discovered every few years in established food additives. At least ten chemicals listed as recently as 1956 by the National Academy of Science in *The Use of Chemical Additives in Food Processing* are currently suspected of being cancer-causing agents. These include a cheese preservative (8-Hydroxyquinilone), a flavoring agent for root beer (safrole), a cheese stabilizer (carboxymethyl cellulose), and several coal-tar dyes. Perhaps the worst offenders are the dyes, notably Yellow AB and OB, which were used for decades to color butter, cheese, cake, candy, cookies, drugs, and cosmetics. When ten commercial samples of these food colors were analyzed by Walter D. Conway and Elizabeth J. Lethco, of the National Cancer Institute, they were found to contain very large residues of beta-naphthalamine, ranging from a low of 76 to a high of 908 parts per million.

Although recent legislation stipulates that no carcinogen may be used as a food additive, there are several noteworthy exceptions. Lead arsenate, for example, is still employed as an insecticide in orchards and vineyards. Residues of the compound (usually 7 parts per million) are allowed to remain on such common fruits as apples, pears, plums, peaches, cherries, and grapes. "It has been known for many years that exposure to arsenicals produces a certain type of cancer of the skin," Francis E. Ray, director of the University of Florida's Cancer Research Laboratory, told the Delaney Committee. "More recent evidence is that inhalation of arsenic dust

—and sprays—may cause cancer of the lungs. It is possible that other types of internal cancer may be caused by the long-continued ingestion of so-called non-toxic doses of arsenicals." Ray declared that the use of arsenicals on crops "should be prohibited." The demand, although reiterated by many outstanding cancer specialists, has largely been ignored.

"While not within the scope of this investigation," Ray added, "it may be mentioned that female sex hormones [estrogens] have been incorporated into cosmetics. These hormones have been shown to induce cancer in female animals when administered for a prolonged period. Their use in cosmetics should be prohibited." * Thus far, however, no action has been taken to forbid the use of estrogens in facial creams. In fact, the use of synthetic hormones has been extended, not reduced. For example, synthetic hormones, notably stilbestrol, are now added to 85 per cent of the cattle feed produced in the United States. A woman who purchases a cosmetic that contains hormones exercises a choice, but a consumer who acquires residues of stilbestrol in meat belongs to a "captive" population whose wishes have not been consulted by food producers or government agencies. Whether the stilbestrol fed to livestock makes its way into meat has been the subject of heated controversy. Regulations prepared by the F.D.A. stipulate that daily feedings of the drug should not exceed 10 milligrams for steers and 2 milligrams for sheep. According to the F.D.A., residues of stilbestrol are avoided when hormone-containing feed is withdrawn forty-eight hours before slaughtering. Actually, the evidence for this claim is equivocal. Although F. O. Gossett and his co-workers found that residues did not

* The most commonly used estrogens in facial creams are estradiol and estrone. Hueper warns that although estrogenic creams are applied to the skin, they occasionally produce systemic effects.

appear in meat when the F.D.A.'s regulations were followed, C. W. Turner detected traces of stilbestrol in the
lungs and kidneys of animals slaughtered forty-four hours
after the prescribed 10-milligram dosages had been withdrawn.

Experimental work on mice by a group of researchers
at the National Cancer Institute indicates that stilbestrol
is a highly potent drug. Practically all the mice that had
received a subcutaneous implantation of 1 milligram of
the synthetic hormone acquired tumors of the testicles
within seven months. When the pellet was removed after
eight weeks, no gross tumors developed, but when it was
reimplanted twenty-four weeks later, the incidence of
tumors rose sharply, as though the pellet had never been
removed. The effect of a brief stimulus is never lost; exposure to stilbestrol seems to be cumulative.

Thousands of man-made chemicals with undeter-
mined properties enter our food supply, water, and air.
Some may be co-carcinogens; these lack significant cancer-causing properties of their own but increase the
potency of known carcinogenic agents. Others may be
weak carcinogens whose cancer-causing effects are additive and synergistic. Any such carcinogens and co-
carcinogens would escape the attention of the researcher
unless they were brought into combination with one
another. But this is a rare experimental procedure.
"Potential carcinogenic contaminants," Hueper warns,
"also may be introduced into foodstuffs if vegetables,
fruits, fish, oysters, and livestock are grown on soil or in
water polluted with known carcinogens, such as radioactive matter, arsenicals, selenium and polycyclic hydrocarbons contained in ship fuel oils, since these chemicals
may be taken up and stored by the vegetable and animal
matter growing in such contaminated media. . . . There
exists also the possibility that originally noncarcinogenic

additives and contaminants may interreact with each other or with food constituents and form new compounds possessing carcinogenic properties in the foodstuffs. They may be produced under the influence of processing procedures or during the preparation of food in the kitchen. Plastics used as wrapping material, sausage skins and coating material of fruits, cheese, meat, butter, and can linings may carry similar hazards."

These are not irresponsible vagaries. A number of chlorinated hydrocarbons, such as DDT, seem to have mild tumor-inducing effects. Nearly all insecticides are dissolved in petroleum distillates, many of which are also suspected of being carcinogens. Crude and semi-refined paraffin waxes, from which cosmetics and food containers are made, have carcinogenic properties and, in some cases, contain residues of highly potent cancer-causing substances. Hans L. Falk, Paul Kotin, and Adele Miller found that the protein in ordinary milk could eluate, or extract, hydrocarbons from the wax coating of their containers. The investigators had deliberately impregnated the wax with these hydrocarbons so that the eluant properties of milk could be tested. "However," they write, "an analysis of several dairy waxes revealed the presence of a small amount of 1,2,5,6-dibenzanthracene of the order of one part per million." Dibenzanthracene, a highly potent carcinogen, appears as an impurity in many semi-refined paraffins.

It is difficult to specify all the potential hazards to public health that are created by saturating man's environment with poorly tested, exotic chemicals. Many cancers are stealthy; they develop slowly and imperceptibly. Decades may pass before mistakes committed today finally bear their malignant fruit; we may pay a heavy price in human life, not so much as a result of brief exposures to a few potent carcinogens as because of the exposure of millions of individuals to small quantities of "harmless" compounds over long periods. The potent carcinogens "by their very strength are almost sure to be discovered clinically," Kotin writes. "In essence, a strong carcinogen identifies itself by the very circumstances which aroused suspicion in the first place. It is assuredly the less potent carcinogens that seem to be more important in human cancer, and it is these that provide the real problem for evaluation."

ENVIRONMENT AND LUNG CANCER

THE INCIDENCE of one kind of malignant tumor, lung cancer, has begun to increase at an appalling rate. "A century ago, Rokitansky of Vienna, the most experienced pathologist of his time, considered lung cancer a rarity" Peller observes. "In other and older books with detailed descriptions of cancer, the lungs are not mentioned at all, whereas cancer of the larynx and of the nose are discussed. Fifty years ago, in hospitals, larynx cancer in the United States was 1.5 times as frequent as lung cancer. In 1947-48, 9 per cent of all fatal cancers, namely 18,144, developed in the respiratory organs and only 1,870 of them originated in the larynx. The number of recorded lung cancers is rising more rapidly than that of any other subgroup."

Although it could be claimed that before X rays were discovered many lung cancers were mistaken for other respiratory disorders, the opinion of an experienced, conscientious medical man such as Rokitansky cannot be ignored. If lung cancer had been a common disease a century ago, it would not have been regarded as a medical curiosity by many of the leading pathologists of the day. During the last five decades the incidence of lung cancer increased at a startling rate, and today the disease is very common. In 1914 seven white American males per million died of lung cancer. By 1956, this figure had reached 284, a fortyfold increase in less than half a century.

It is difficult to attribute these higher figures to improvements in diagnostic technique. By the 1930's, X rays were being used extensively in the United States and biopsies involving the microscopic analysis of cancerous tissue were frequently performed. Nevertheless, the number of deaths from lung cancer among American males rose steadily after 1930 until it had increased 500 per cent by 1951. Even more conclusive evidence against the "diagnostic improvement" argument is supplied by data from the Copenhagen Tuberculosis Station in Denmark. "In a tuberculosis referral service, used extensively by local physicians, where diagnostic standards and procedures including systematic bronchoscopy remained virtually unchanged between 1941 and 1950, the lung-cancer prevalence rate among male examinees increased at a rate comparable to that recorded by the Danish cancer registry for the total male population," Jerome Cornfield and his colleagues observe in an excellent review of the lung-cancer problem. "This can be regarded as evidence that the reported increase in Danish incidence is not due to diagnostic changes."

It is equally difficult to attribute the rise in the number of cases of lung cancer to the increased longevity of the population. Whatever may be the factors that account for the high incidence of cancer in older people, careful study has shown, Cornfield observes, that "only one sixth of the over-all increase in lung-cancer mortality among

males in the United States (from 4 to 24 deaths per
100,000 males between 1930 and 1951) could be attributed to an aging population. Similar findings have been
presented for England and Wales. . . . Allowance for increased average age of the population could account for
only half this rise in lung-cancer mortality, with a 24-
fold difference between 1900 and 1953."

Nor is it a convincing argument that the rise in
deaths from lung cancer is due to cancers that begin in
one part of the body and later migrate to the lungs.
Autopsies have proved this to be a fallacy. Cornfield and
his associates reviewed thirteen series of such autopsies,
the first begun early in the present century and the last
completed in the 1950's. These autopsies support the
claim that mortality from primary lung cancer has increased sharply during the past fifty years.

The inescapable conclusion seems to be that the
rising incidence of lung cancer is due to recent changes
in man's environment and manner of life. What are the
changes? The majority of American biostatisticians and
cancer specialists believe that cases of lung cancer are
multiplying because of the increased consumption of
cigarettes, and they have collected an enormous amount
of statistical evidence to support this belief. "Twenty-two
. . . studies of smoking in relation to lung cancer have
now been carried out independently in eight different
countries," notes E. C. Hammond, of the American Cancer
Society. "In every one of these, a far larger proportion
of smokers (particularly heavy cigarette smokers) was
found among lung cancer patients than among people
without this disease. This has been shown for both men
and women." Hammond adds that "similar studies have
shown an association between smoking and cancer of
the buccal cavity, cancer of the larynx, cancer of the

bladder, coronary artery disease (the most common form of heart disease), and Buerger's disease (a circulatory disease of the extremities)."

Thus far the most important attempt to correlate the rising incidence of lung cancer with increased smoking has been the survey made under the direction of E. C. Hammond and Daniel Horn for the American Cancer Society. The society mobilized 22,000 volunteers as researchers, and asked each of them to have about ten men between fifty and sixty-nine years of age complete a questionnaire on their smoking habits. Precautions were taken to query only individuals who were not seriously ill, who apparently were not suffering from lung cancer, and with whom the research volunteers enjoyed some measure of personal contact, so that thorough follow-ups could be made. Nearly 190,000 acceptable questionnaires were obtained during the first half of 1952. Almost 188,000 were followed up by the volunteers through October 1955. A careful study of the death certificates of about 12,000 men who died during the three-year period yielded remarkable results. Comparing smokers with non-smokers in the same age groups, Hammond and Horn found that the general death rate was 9 per cent higher for occasional smokers, 12 per cent higher for pipe smokers, and 68 per cent higher for cigarette smokers. The death rate for cigarette smokers increased progressively with the quantity of cigarettes smoked, nearly doubling with a rise in consumption from a half pack to two or more packs daily. It was found that the incidence of lung cancer among cigarette smokers was almost twice as high as it was among non-smokers. Comparing moderate smokers (a half pack daily) and heavy smokers (two or more packs daily) with non-smokers, Hammond and Horn found that the ratio of death from lung cancer soared to 17 to 1 and 60 to 1, respectively.

Those who maintain that there is no relationship between lung cancer and smoking have been placed in an
untenable position. At first it was held that there was no
direct evidence to implicate tobacco tars in cancer in
animals. This contention was shaken when at least six
different laboratories reported that such tars induced skin
cancer in mice. It was then claimed that although tobacco tars may cause skin cancer in mice, it had not
been shown that they could cause lung cancer in mice,
men, or any other species of animal. This argument is
difficult to sustain, at least as far as men are concerned.
In a co-operative project initiated in 1954 under the
direction of two leading American pathologists, Oscar
Auerbach and Arthur Sout, the entire breathing apparatus
was systematically removed from all individuals autop-
sied at the Veterans Hospital in East Orange, New Jersey,
and at eleven hospitals in New York State. The investigators were able to obtain reliable histories of smoking on
402 of the subjects, all of them white males, 63 of whom
had died of lung cancer. After preparing nearly 20,000
usable slides of lung tissue from the 402 subjects and
carefully examining each slide under the microscope, the
pathologists found that tissue abnormalities (changes in
the epithelium) appeared in only 16.8 per cent of the
slides from non-smokers, in 92.3 per cent of those from
light smokers, in 97.4 per cent of those from moderate
smokers (a half pack to a pack daily), and in nearly 100
per cent of the slides from those who smoked more than a
pack daily. The changes in the lung tissue from atypical,
potentially cancerous cells to invasive, cancerous cells
increased with the average intake of cigarettes. Focusing their attention on all the subjects who had died from
causes other than lung cancer, Auerbach and Sout found
that 22.6 per cent of the slides from heavy smokers had
atypical cells and 11.4 per cent had cancerous cells. On

the other hand, only 0.2 per cent of the slides from non-smokers had atypical cells and none had cancerous cells.

However, disinterested critics of the theory that smoking and lung cancer are related have performed a very useful function. By looking for other factors besides smoking, they have drawn a great deal of attention to the role that air pollution plays in producing the disease. The relationship between air pollution and lung cancer has largely been ignored despite evidence that lung-cancer rates are higher in cities than they are in rural areas. But as more research is done, zealots on both sides in the lung-cancer controversy are moving toward a more balanced position. An impressive amount of statistical evidence implicates air pollution as well as smoking in the rising incidence of lung cancer. White South African males, for example, are probably the heaviest smokers of packaged cigarettes in the world, and the number of deaths from lung cancer among them has increased from 11.7 per 100,000 in 1947 to 24.6 in 1956. But South Africa presents an interesting opportunity for statistical research. The country has acquired a large number of British immigrants, most of whom came from English cities with heavily polluted air. Is the incidence of lung cancer higher among British immigrants than among native-born South Africans? After a careful statistical study, Geoffrey Dean, of the Provincial Hospital in Port Elizabeth, South Africa, established that in the forty-five-to-sixty-four age group, deaths from lung cancer were 44 per cent higher among a group of British male immigrants than among native-born males. The incidence of the disease rose with the age at which immigration occurred, indicating that longer residence in England increased the possibility of dying from lung cancer. The difference in the death rate between native-born and British-born males could not be explained by differences in cigarette brands; the two groups smoked very much the same brands. But Dean's data in no way indicate that prolonged smoking is not hazardous. On the contrary, the steadily rising rate of death from lung cancer observed in both groups of males supports the contention that cigarette consumption plays a major role in causing the disease.

The air over the metropolitan districts of the United States and Europe contains a large variety of known carcinogens. Perhaps the most potent of these agents are the so-called polycyclic hydrocarbons, such as benzpyrene and anthracene. By painting the skin of mice with benzpyrene three times weekly for six months, E. L. Wynder and his co-workers were able to produce cancers in nearly half the animals. An individual who smokes a pack of cigarettes a day acquires about 60 micrograms (millionths of a gram) of benzpyrene a year. If he lives in Helena, Montana, he inhales 0.8 micrograms of benzpyrene from the air annually; in Los Angeles, he inhales 20; in Detroit, 110; and in London, 320. That is, he acquires the equivalent of the benzpyrene in a third of a pack of cigarettes daily merely by breathing the air in Los Angeles, the benzpyrene in nearly two packs from the air in Detroit, and the benzpyrene in five packs from the air in London. It should not be surprising to learn that death rates for lung cancer among males in England are more than twice those in the United States.

Kotin found that when an efficient automobile engine revolves 500 times per minute for one minute, it produces a gasoline exhaust containing 235 micrograms of benzpyrene. When the engine is accelerated to 3,500 revolutions per minute, the amount of benzpyrene in the exhaust decreases to 10 micrograms. A congested thoroughfare cluttered with idling or slow-moving motor vehicles is a hazard to human lungs. Individuals who spend a large part of their time in such areas, irrespective of the particular metropolis in which they live, are likely to acquire a lifetime dosage of benzpyrene that is thousands of times greater than the amount required to produce cancer in mice.

In addition to smoking and air pollution, socioeconomic factors have been found to play a role in the incidence of lung cancer. It is a tempting hypothesis that susceptibility to the disease is increased by poor nutrition, economic insecurity, and low physical resistance. "The existence of other important lung-cancer effects associated with such characteristics as socioeconomic class cannot be questioned," Cornfield and his co-workers state. "Cohart found that the poorest economic class had a 40 per cent higher lung-cancer incidence than the remaining population of New Haven, Connecticut. Results of the 10-city morbidity survey [by Dorn and Cutler] have revealed a sharp gradient in lung-cancer incidence, by income class, for white males, which is consistent with Cohart's findings. Since cigarette smoking is not inversely related to socioeconomic status, we can agree with Cohart '. . . that important environmental factors other than cigarette smoking exist that contribute to the causation of lung cancer.' These and other findings are convincing evidence for multiple causes of lung cancer. It is obviously untenable to regard smoking of tobacco as the sole cause of lung cancer." *

What can we learn from these studies? There no longer seems to be any doubt that the rising incidence of lung cancer is due to recent changes in our synthetic environment. So compelling are the data now at hand that

* This conclusion is apparently shared by Hammond and Wynder, who not only were co-authors of Cornfield's report but also played an outstanding role in focusing public attention on the hazards of cigarette smoking.

virtually the entire scientific community has been obliged to accept this conclusion. One can only wonder why it was not accepted earlier. The growing incidence of lung cancer was noted as early as 1929 in the German *Journal for Cancer Research* by Fritz Lickint, who thought that the disease was related to smoking. In 1932 the same relationship was explored by W. D. McNally in the *American Journal of Cancer Research*. Lickint and McNally were followed by other investigators, including Alton Ochsner, who wrote on the subject in 1941, but the scientific community remained largely unmoved. More than a decade passed before Hammond and Horn finally presented the problem of the relationship between lung cancer and smoking in a form that was too compelling to be ignored. Until then, the rise in the number of cases of lung cancer was generally attributed to genetic factors or to increased longevity.

It should be noted that it has taken many years for an obvious link between environmental changes and the rising incidence of a major disease to gain wide acceptance among scientists. Because of its highly charged social, economic, and political implications, man's environment is an arena that scientific research tends to enter with reluctance. There is a strong disposition to probe heredity, a more neutral field, or to dismiss grave problems of disease as the consequence of greater longevity. But now the evidence of the direct connection between the rising incidence of lung cancer and changes in man's environment has affected this traditional approach profoundly. We now have good reasons for questioning whether any type of cancer need burden mankind as heavily as it does today. We have begun to take a closer look at the irrationalities in our synthetic environment. Perhaps we shall begin to eliminate them.

But we cannot wait indefinitely before making man's

environment and manner of life more rational. Mortality from cancer is rising steadily. In the United States, known deaths from the disease increased 22 per cent between 1940 and 1959, an increase that can scarcely be accounted for by any monumental improvements in diagnostic technique. Recently a survey of 610 women by the New York City Cancer Committee showed that more than a third had symptoms suggestive of malignant tumors or a pre-cancerous condition. None of the women was more than forty-two years old. Robert A. Loberfeld, vice-president of the committee, is quoted in a news item as describing the situation as "shocking." Cancer has even reached epidemic proportions. At the Fourth National Cancer Conference, in September 1960, Lester Breslow reported that "tens of thousands" of trout in western hatcheries suddenly acquired liver cancers. Apparently the disease was "associated with a new type of diet," not with a virus.

"Technological changes affecting man's environment are being introduced at such a rapid rate and with so little control that it is a wonder man has thus far escaped the type of cancer epidemic occurring this year among the trout," Breslow told his colleagues. "Or have we? Lung cancer is not too dissimilar except that the time period is decades, not weeks. If community air pollution of the types now prevailing or being introduced by technological changes is proved to be a causative factor in lung cancer, we would be dealing with exposure of millions of people. New pollutants are frequently added nowadays to community air through changes in industrial process, fuel composition and the like. They are added for reasons of economy or efficiency in industry or transportation—essentially the same reasons given for changing the diet of the fish. It is not inconceivable that although cigarette smoking has been the major factor in the lung cancer epidemic during the first half of the 20th century, some form of community air pollution could be responsible for an even larger epidemic of the disease during the second half of the 20th century."

Radiation and Human Health

THE EFFECTS OF RADIATION

IT IS HARDLY necessary to emphasize that since the explosion of a nuclear weapon at Alamogordo, New Mexico, in July 1945, ionizing radiation has become the most serious threat to man's survival. If nuclear weapons are further developed or increased in number, it is quite conceivable that a future war will virtually extinguish human life. Grave as this danger may be, ionizing radiation is associated with a number of subtle hazards that warrant equal public concern. "Today . . . sources of ionizing radiation are rapidly becoming more and more widely used," observes a team of radiation specialists for the U. S. Public Health Service. "Each atomic reactor produces the radioactive equivalent of hundreds of pounds of radium. Radioactive substances are used in increasing numbers of hospitals, industries, and research establishments. X-ray machines are encountered in tuberculosis surveys, in shoe stores, in physicians' offices and in foundries. Potentially, ionizing radiation has come to affect the environment of every member of the community."

Radioactive elements are among the most lethal toxicants in man's environment. As little as four micrograms (one seven-millionth of an ounce) of radium is capable of producing cancer in man years after lodging in his bones. Not all radioactive elements are dangerous in the same way as radium. Some are distributed differently in the body and are not retained for long periods; others, although retained for years, emit different kinds of radiation. Strontium-90, for example, is rated about one tenth as lethal as radium, although it, too, lodges primarily in the bones. Attempts to compare the potency of the two elements in quantitative terms, however, can be somewhat misleading. Radium causes biological damage through the emission of alpha particles, whereas strontium-90 is hazardous to living things because it is an energetic emitter of beta particles. "Leukemia has been observed to occur in radium patients, though not as a prominent phenomenon," observes W. F. Neuman, of the University of Rochester. "Leukemia is, however, a common finding in people who have suffered irradiation of the bone marrow or of the whole body. Since the beta rays from strontium-90 are more penetrating than the alpha rays from radium, a greater proportion of the rays from strontium-90 will penetrate into the marrow." It is quite possible that, for individuals prone to leukemia, strontium-90 poses hazards in addition to those that would be expected on the basis of criteria derived from experiences with radium.

To gain a clear understanding of the various kinds of radiation and their biological effects, it will be useful to review briefly some elementary concepts of atomic physics. Radioactivity is produced by changes that occur within the nucleus of an atom. These changes either directly or indirectly involve two nuclear particles, the neutron and the proton. The number of neutrons (electrically neutral particles) and protons (positively charged particles) in an atomic nucleus determines the species to which the atom belongs. Carbon-12 and carbon-13, for example, have six and seven neutrons, respectively, and are called isotopes of the element carbon. Every carbon atom, however, has six protons in its nucleus and an equal number of external electrons (negatively charged particles), which can be thought of as "revolving" around the nucleus like planets in a miniature solar system. Similarly, all hydrogen atoms have one proton and one planetary electron, whereas hydrogen-2 and hydrogen-3 have one and two neutrons, respectively. When carbon and hydrogen combine to form hydrocarbons, the nuclear particles (protons and neutrons) of the two elements are not affected by the combination. The chemical reaction of carbon and hydrogen is determined by the arrangement of their planetary electrons. Each element can be separated from the other without any loss of its original identity and without producing ionizing radiation. On the other hand, if carbon were to gain or lose any protons, it would become an entirely different element. Gains or losses in the number of protons may occur when a neutron is converted into a proton, when a proton is converted into a neutron, and, of course, when a proton together with a neutron is emitted from the nucleus of an atom. These changes and the various energy adjustments that occur within the nucleus produce ionizing radiation.

The more familiar elements that make up the earth do not undergo nuclear changes spontaneously. Their nuclei are extremely stable. A few elements, however, such as uranium, radium, and polonium, have unstable nuclei. They emit particles and eventually break down into more stable elements. Radium, which is derived from the decay of uranium, disintegrates into radon by emitting two protons and two neutrons. Decay continues through a series of radioactive daughter products until the atom becomes lead. The two protons and two neutrons emitted by the radium atom remain together and constitute an alpha particle. Streams of these neutron-proton groups, or alpha "rays," are emitted from radium nuclei at velocities of about 44,000 miles per second. In addition, radium emits gamma rays, and several daughter products of the element emit beta rays. Beta rays are streams of electrons and positrons (the positive counterparts of electrons); they travel at varying speeds, sometimes approaching the speed of light (186,000 miles per second). Gamma rays are physically the same as X rays, the difference in name arising from the difference in the sources of emission.* It takes 1,600 years for half a given quantity of radium to disintegrate into radon. Another 1,600 years must pass before the remaining quantity of radium is halved again. As this process goes on indefinitely, always leaving a remainder to be halved each 1,600 years, some radium will remain for an immensely long period. By the same token, by adding radioactive substances to his environment, man increases the amount that will remain indefinitely, whether the half-life of an element is 5,900 years (carbon-14) or 28 years

* X radiation is produced when a fast-moving, free electron collides violently with an atomic nucleus and loses part of its surrounding electric field. Unlike gamma radiation, however, X radiation does not involve any energy adjustments within atomic nuclei.

(strontium-90). Although man can create radioactive elements such as strontium-90, there is nothing he can do to reduce their radioactivity. Radiation continues undisturbed, and is diminished only with the passage of time.

What effects do alpha, beta, and gamma rays produce in living tissues? Although the long-range effects of low-level radiation on animals and man are very much in dispute, there seems to be little doubt about the harmful changes radiation produces in cells. Radiation particles have been compared to bullets tearing into an organism, but the damage they cause depends upon the number of particles that reach the tissues. The particles interact with many of the atoms that make up our cells, either causing electrons to leave their orbits (ionization) or exciting combinations of atoms (molecules) to a point where they break apart. The resulting damage may be minor and easily repaired; on the other hand, it may be serious and permanent. Irradiated germ cells may one day give rise to harmful mutations, and irradiated body cells may take the first step toward the development of cancer. An individual exposed to large dosages of radiation may exhibit symptoms of "radiation sickness"—nausea, vomiting, loss of hair, progressive weakness, and hemorrhages. Severe irradiation of the entire body damages the blood-forming organs in man and higher animals, often claiming life within several weeks after exposure. If the whole body is exposed to very high levels of radiation, there will be widespread destruction of the intestinal tract and nerve cells. In such cases, death is certain to occur within a few days after exposure.

Quantities of radiation are usually expressed in terms of rads and roentgens.* A rad denotes the quantity

* These units are used in most of the works cited in this discussion. During the past few years, however, the rad has been steadily

of radiation an individual absorbs; a roentgen denotes the amount of radiation (ordinarily X radiation) to which he is exposed. For the purposes of this discussion, no significant distinction need be made between the two units. A single rad *or* roentgen can be thought of as giving rise to about 1,000 ionizations in a single cell. An individual normally receives a total dosage of 3 to 5 roentgens from natural background radiation during the first thirty years of his life. Background radiation comes from cosmic rays, radioactivity in rocks, and radioactive elements in food and water. It constitutes the radiation to which man has evidently adapted himself over long periods of biological evolution. Although background radiation will vary in amount from one locale to another, the absolute quantities involved are ordinarily very small. A man living at sea level usually absorbs about 30 millirads (30 thousandths of a rad) of cosmic radiation a year. A man living at 5,000 feet above sea level is likely to absorb about 70 millirads annually. An individual who moves from sea level to a height of 5,000 feet will thus raise his absorption of cosmic radiation by little more than a rad during a thirty-year period. A man who remains behind at sea level may well acquire more than that amount in certain parts of his body, by having a tooth X-rayed, for example. In fact, a series of dental X rays will supply his jaw and neck with a larger amount of radiation than they are likely to acquire from natural background sources in the greater part of a normal life span.

When X rays are used for diagnostic or therapeutic purposes, the good they do outweighs the harm. Diagnostic X rays are usually directed at limited areas of the body, a form of exposure that is far less hazardous than

supplanted by the rem (*r*oentgen *e*quivalent *m*an) in discussions of the effects of radiation on humans. The terms "rem" and "rad" signify identical values for exposure to beta and gamma radiation.

irradiation of the whole body. However, despite recent claims to the contrary, there is no conclusive evidence that small doses of radiation are harmless. Although some research workers have reported that very low levels of radiation (5 roentgens or less per week) increase longevity in animals, others working with similar doses of radiation have found that the life span is shortened. In the cases in which increases in longevity were reported, the last animals to die were generally non-irradiated control animals. If radiation had any "beneficial" effect, it was that it seemed to reduce the death rate of irradiated animals in early age groups, but the maximum life span of the animals was shortened.*

There seems to be very little ambiguity, however, about the genetic effects of radiation. All the facts at hand indicate that any increase in the amount of radiation received by a large population produces a rise in the occurrence of harmful mutations. Nor do we have to rely exclusively on experiments with animals to acquire statistically significant evidence to support this conclusion. A study made by John T. Gentry and his colleagues in the New York State Department of Health suggests that areas with relatively high concentrations of radioactive rock are correlated with a high incidence of congenitally malformed children—many, perhaps most, of whose defects are believed to be caused by defective genes. By working primarily with statistics compiled from a million and a quarter birth certificates in New York State

* In the opinion of Alex Comfort, one of England's foremost authorities on the aging process in animals and man, the increase in longevity produced by low-level radiation "is due partly to the slight physiological stimulus arising from 'stress' and partly to the fact that radiation at these low levels does more harm to parasites of various kinds than to the animals infected with them. In any case, the life extension is seen only in animal colonies where the survival curve is suboptimal. Among animals that are well cared for, radiation, if it has any visible effect, shortens life."

(exclusive of New York City), Gentry found that the over-all incidence of congenital malformation amounted to 12.9 per 1,000 live births in areas of the state which seemed to have the least amount of geologic radioactivity. The incidence of congenital malformation for areas which seemed to have the highest amount of geologic radioactivity was 17.5—a difference of nearly 40 per cent. New York State, it should be noted, is not particularly radioactive; field measurements of background radiation were found to lie mainly in the range of 2.1 to 3.2 roentgens per thirty-year period. Additional evidence that the rate of malformation is influenced by the radioactivity of the geologic environment appears in a preliminary nation-wide study by Jack Kratchman and Douglas Grahn, of the U. S. Atomic Energy Commission. By grouping county and state mortality data according to the geologic provinces of the United States, Kratchman and Grahn found that "mortality incidence from malformation may be higher in those geologic provinces . . . that contain major uranium ore deposits, uraniferous waters or helium concentrations."

These studies are a reminder that man is probably far more sensitive to radiation than has generally been supposed. Although the living matter that surrounds the nucleus of a cell can often absorb a great deal of radiation without being significantly harmed, the nucleus itself is highly vulnerable. Theodore T. Puck and his co-workers at the University of Colorado Medical Center have recently shown that visible damage can be inflicted on chromosomes (the strands in the nucleus of the cell that carry the genes) with as little as 20 to 25 roentgens. The genetic apparatus of an ordinary body cell "thus shows extraordinary sensitivity to radiation," Puck observes. "Calculation indicates that the ionization of not more than a few hundred atoms within or around the space occupied by the chromosome may be sufficient to produce a visible break. It seems probable that an even greater number of lesions may occur and remain invisible, either because they are submicroscopic or because they become resealed before they are expanded."

If radiation is increased to 50 roentgens, many cells soon lose the ability to reproduce, although they do not necessarily die. The nuclear material of the cell may be damaged beyond recovery, but the cytoplasm surrounding the nucleus survives and performs the essential functions of life. Instead of reproducing, the cells continue to ob-sorb nutriment and grow until they reach enormous size. They become so-called "giant cells," seven to ten times larger than a cell that has not been irradiated. Irradia-tion of the whole body with 400 to 500 roentgens is fatal to half the human beings so exposed, apparently be-cause over 99 per cent of the body's reproducing cells lose the ability to multiply normally. Individuals who receive lethal dosages of radiation may live for weeks after ex-posure, but the body's inability to form a sufficient num-ber of red and white blood cells eventually leads to death from anemia or infection.

Children are probably more sensitive to radiation than adults, and the fetus appears to be more sensitive than the child. Radiation not only has a selective effect upon different parts of a cell; it does the greatest damage to those cells that have a high rate of reproduction. It seems to be most harmful during those stages of life at which metabolism is at its peak, notably the years of growth. Sensitivity varies markedly from individual to individual and from one organ of the body to another. A large whole-body dose of radiation from which some individuals recover with a self-limiting case of "radiation sickness" may lead in others to permanent damage and death. If concentrated on the hand, the same dose may produce nothing more than a radiation burn. Directed at the abdominal area, however, it will often cause serious damage and marked physiological reactions.

Finally, there are different kinds of radiation and various emitters of radiation. The effects produced by all forms of radiation are ordinarily reducible to the amount of ionization they produce. But each form of radiation has distinctive features of its own. The alpha particle is the "heavy artillery shell" of ionizing radiation. As it is made up of two protons joined with two neutrons (actually a nucleus of the element helium), an alpha particle has about 7,300 times the mass of the lighter, faster beta particle. The penetrating power of alpha rays is very limited; they can be stopped by a thin sheet of paper. But although alpha particles do not penetrate very far into living tissue, they score a large number of "direct hits" on atoms. An irradiated cell is damaged more severely by alpha particles than by other forms of radiation, although fewer cells are irradiated by an alpha emitter. If the alpha particle had the penetrating power possessed by beta and gamma rays, it would be extremely destructive to living things.

Beta particles travel about 100 times farther than alpha particles. Whereas alpha particles seldom pass beyond the outer, dead layer of the skin, the free, fast-moving electrons and positrons that constitute beta radiation penetrate for about a quarter of an inch into living matter. Gamma rays and X rays will pass readily through a large organism; they reach the innermost recesses of the body and injure highly sensitive tissues, but they produce only about one twentieth of the damage inflicted on cells by alpha particles.

As gamma rays are physically the same as X rays, we might say that most of the effects produced in man by gamma radiation are due to the widespread use of X-ray equipment. Alpha and primary beta radiations are carried to man's vital organs by radioactive elements.* X-ray equipment can be turned on and off; thus, exposure to X radiation need not be continuous or uncontrolled. But radioactive isotopes cannot be "turned off." Once they combine with the skeleton and the soft tissues of the body, they are no longer within human control. Like the nutrients that sustain life and growth, many radioactive elements become part of the organism. The body tends to use radium and strontium-90, for example, the same way that it employs calcium, although it shows a preference for the latter. Radium and strontium-90 migrate to the mineral part of the skeleton, where the rate of metabolic activity is relatively low, and they bombard bone matter and highly sensitive bone marrow with alpha and beta particles for a long period of time. The body does not discriminate between radioactive and stable carbon isotopes. Carbon-14 appears in every kind of tissue, including germ cells, and irradiates the area in which it lodges with beta particles.

In the field of radiobiology, it is very imprudent to make ironclad generalizations that are likely to affect the well-being of large populations. The field is beset with so many uncertainties that scientific opinion can be expected to differ on nearly every issue but the "need for further research." The public, in turn, would probably acknowledge this need with tranquillity if the problems of radiation were confined to the laboratory. But they are

* The word "primary" is used because beta radiation induces gamma radiation in much the same way that a stream of electrons striking a metal target produces X rays. Gamma radiation, in turn, by imparting energy to the planetary electrons of atoms, causes them to leave their orbits. The free electrons behave like a beta ray. Thus, a short-lived series of radiations, alternating between beta and gamma rays, could extend the range of biological damage to tissues that might not ordinarily be reached by the primary beta ray.

not. X-ray machines are now part of the equipment of every physician and dentist; the devices have become indispensable in medical practice. Radioactive isotopes are used widely in laboratories, hospitals, and industry. Nuclear weapons tests have discharged radioactive debris into the soil, water, and atmosphere, and nuclear reactors are annually producing huge quantities of highly radioactive wastes. The experimental animals needed for further research currently include all of humanity, and the modern radiation laboratory encompasses the entire earth. But many serious questions have been left unanswered. Are we using radiation with the caution and respect it deserves? To what extent have we contaminated the environment? In what direction are we going? Unless these questions are answered frankly and existing abuses corrected, the data acquired by further research may well prove to be of academic importance.

THE PROBLEMS OF X RADIATION

X RAYS WERE THE FIRST form of ionizing radiation to be deliberately produced by man, and in the United States and western Europe they now constitute the radiation to which he is most heavily exposed. Many people of all ages and all walks of life are given routine X rays during periodic medical and dental examinations. Moreover, exposure to X rays has been increasing steadily over the past three decades. According to data gathered by the National Advisory Committee on Radiation, the annual X-ray dosage received by the average American increased 900 per cent between 1925 and 1955. The radiation he receives from X rays is 135 per cent greater than the radiation he acquires from natural sources. "The continued upward trend exhibited by X-ray data," observes the committee, "suggests the likelihood that the current exposure of the population from X-ray apparatus may increase still further unless appropriate radiation control measures are systematically applied."

Systematic control of X radiation is long overdue. Man-induced radiation has been in use since 1896, the year Roentgen's discovery of X rays attracted world-wide attention, and the effective application of these rays to medical problems antedates World War I. Surprisingly, a good working knowledge of the hazards of X radiation and valuable recommendations for the proper use of X-ray equipment were available shortly after Roentgen's work became well known. Elihu Thomson, after experimenting with the new rays on his little finger, reported a great deal of the data needed to enable radiologists to use X-ray equipment with a reasonable amount of safety. His suggestions were largely ignored. For many years X-ray tubes were employed with little or no shielding, while physicians, in blissful disregard of Thomson's recommendations, often exposed themselves as well as their patients to heavy doses of radiation. By the early 1920's, scores of radiologists had needlessly sacrificed their lives and, in all probability, inflicted a great deal of damage on many of their unsuspecting patients.

To make matters worse, X-ray equipment was rapidly debased into a cosmetic agent and, finally, into a sales-promotion device. It was found that X rays could cause a loss of hair (epilation), an effect that suggested lucrative possibilities. By the 1920's many physicians, beauticians, and self-appointed "epilation specialists" had begun to treat women with radiation for the removal of "superfluous hair." One New York physician, Dr. Albert C. Geyser, developed a "harmless" method of hair removal that involved cumulative dosages of at least 500 roentgens over a twelve-week period of radiation treatment. The method, named the "Tricho System," was very successful, and beauticians trained by Geyser's "Tricho Institute" began operating in many parts of the United States and Canada. It soon became evident, however, that women treated according to the "Tricho System" lost substantially more than unwanted hair. Many individuals acquired radiodermatitis (skin inflammation), severe radiation burns, festering skin ulcers, and, in time, cancer. The "Tricho" story is one of the more tragic episodes in the history of radiation. It is believed that the victims of Geyser's system numbered in the thousands; the exact number of those who suffered latent injury and premature death will never be known.

Although radiation is no longer employed in the American beauty parlor, the use of X-ray equipment to fit shoes still lingers in a number of communities. The equipment is used mainly on the feet of children. As of 1960, the use of the shoe-fitting fluoroscope had been banned in twenty-nine states. Some of the other states regulate the use of the machine, but in a few states there are no restrictions at all. A number of local surveys cited by Schubert and Lapp have shown that the machines are often defective, giving high doses of radiation to both the child and the salesman. The Michigan Department of Health, for example, found shoe-fitting machines that emitted as many as 65 roentgens (r) a minute. A survey in Boston showed that irradiation of the foot ranged from 0.5 to 5.8 r a second.* "For a 22-second exposure, which is commonly used, the feet receive from 10 to 116 r!" Schubert and Lapp write. "Remember, too, that one child

---

* The use of shoe-fitting fluoroscopes has been banned in Boston by state law and is regulated in Michigan.

may have his feet examined many times while trying on different shoes. Similar dosage measurements have been reported by the United States Public Health Service, which states that the average dosages to the children's feet are between 7 r and 14 r per exposure." The amount of scattered radiation that reaches the child's pelvic region and gonads may run as high as 0.2 roentgens for a twenty-second exposure.

Society has found it very difficult to accept the fact that a valuable device can become extremely dangerous if it is used improperly. Schubert and Lapp observe that a major reason why Geyser was not stopped until his "system" had injured a large number of women is that the medical community generally accepted radiation as a form of treatment for minor skin disorders. To this day, many physicians are likely to underestimate the amount of latent damage caused by repeated exposure to X radiation. In some cases, physicians are inclined to use X-ray equipment as freely as they use the stethoscope, and often it is the cost of an X-ray picture rather than the risk of irradiation that keeps the two devices from occupying places of equal importance in routine medical examinations. The physician often feels that there is no danger involved in taking diagnostic X rays; the word "diagnostic" seems to impart benign qualities to radiation. But the need for an X ray does not in any way diminish the effect of exposure; it merely provides a scale on which the hazards of X radiation should be weighed against the hazards of an incomplete and faulty diagnosis.

This requires careful evaluation. A middle-aged man who refuses to be exposed to the small amount of radiation involved in an annual chest X ray carries his fear of radiation to extremes. The risk involved in having an X ray taken is much smaller than the risk involved in permitting a serious lung disease to remain undiagnosed.

Schubert and Lapp estimate that sixty chest X rays taken on a 14-by-17-inch plate without accompanying fluoroscopies will give an individual a cumulative dose of 3 roentgens. With newly developed fast films, exposure is likely to be reduced appreciably. Similarly, a man with marked and prolonged gastrointestinal distress who fails to respond to treatment for benign stomach disorders would be foolhardy if he refused to have X rays taken of his abdominal region. The danger of serious disease would outweigh by far the amount of harm caused by a single series of X rays.

But individuals without medical complaints who are exposed periodically to a large amount of diagnostic radiation might do well to entertain some second thoughts. For example, many large American corporations have established the practice of sending their executives to clinics for annual medical examinations. These examinations take several days to perform and normally include a program of X rays and fluoroscopies of important organs of the body. Schubert and Lapp found that an executive can expect to receive 35 roentgens with each check-up; frequently the dosages reach 50 roentgens. "We grant that the executive is not exposed to total body radiation, which is more serious than localized radiation," they write. "Nevertheless, the most vital organs are exposed and at the very least one may expect a shortening of life span of the exposed individual, especially if the executive receives the x-ray bombardment year after year. We do not deny the valuable data which doctors may gain in the course of x-ray examination, which may lengthen the life span, but we do regard the annual irradiation of 50 r per executive with some degree of apprehension for the individual's future welfare."

A number of radiobiologists believe that certain X rays should not be undertaken unless they are absolutely necessary for the well-being of the patient. A case in point is the pelvic X ray (pelvimetry) of pregnant women. "X-ray pelvimetries have been a relatively common practice for many years—and still is as far as is known," Schubert told a congressional committee holding hearings on radiation in 1959. An estimated 440,000 American women and 100,000 English women were given pelvic X rays annually during the late 1950's. The practice had always aroused a certain amount of concern because of the harmful genetic effects it could produce in later generations, but recent studies show that the hazards may be more immediate. In an extensive survey of deaths from cancer among English and Welsh children, Alice Stewart and her co-workers at Oxford University found a statistical relationship between fetal irradiation and the incidence of cancer among children. The survey, perhaps the most extensive of its kind, covered most of the children who had died of leukemia and other cancers between 1953 and 1955. The data gathered by the investigators show that, among children under ten, the chances of dying from cancer are twice as great for those who were irradiated during the fetal stage.

Moderate enlargement of the thymus gland, a condition for which a large number of children have received radiotherapy, is now regarded as harmless by many medical authorities. Although thymic enlargement is no longer treated with radiation in England, the practice still persists in the United States. C. Lenore Simpson and her co-workers have carefully surveyed about 2,000 such cases in New York State, mainly in Rochester and Buffalo. By comparing the incidence of cancer in treated cases with that in children in the general population, they found nearly a sevenfold increase in cancer among children who had been exposed to high dosages of radiation for thymic enlargement. The number of leukemia cases found by Simpson was nearly ten times higher than the number that would normally have been expected.

It remains to be seen whether most radiobiologists will decide that pelvimetries and thymic irradiation produce cancer in children. The evidence is not altogether clear-cut. Several later surveys of a more limited nature have reported findings that conflict with the results obtained by Stewart and Simpson, whereas other surveys support them. The results seem to vary with the methods used and the communities studied. The Stewart and Simpson surveys, however, have unearthed statistical probabilities that are far too high to be dismissed lightly. Although these probabilities can be expected to vary with the techniques of the radiologists in different communities and medical institutions, there seems to be little reason to doubt the validity of the findings of Stewart and Simpson.

Physicians have observed that many children with thyroid cancer received radiation around the head and neck during infancy and early childhood. George Crile, of the Cleveland Clinic Foundation, for example, reports that in 18 cases treated by his clinic, the parents of 14 were asked whether their children had been exposed to X rays in the general area of the thyroid gland. Only 3 had not received radiation. The remaining 11 had histories of radiotherapy for enlargement of the thymus gland and lymph nodes, for eczema, and for other disorders. "In the 15 years between 1924 and 1939," Crile notes, "at a time when many more operations on the thyroid were being done at the Cleveland Clinic than are being done today, no children with cancers of the thyroid were seen. Only three were seen between 1939 and 1950, and between 1950 and 1958 there were 15 cases. The question immediately arises as to whether the increasing incidence of cancer of the thyroid in children is the result of an increase in the use of radiation therapy in infancy and early childhood." Crile notes that factors other than radiation may account for the rise in thyroid cancer among children but adds that "the increasing incidence of cancer of the thyroid in recent years suggests that an environmental factor such as radiation is involved."

Many individuals are still exposed to large dosages of X radiation for what are essentially cosmetic purposes. Localized eczemas, warts, and childhood birthmarks that are likely to disappear spontaneously after a few years have in many cases been heavily irradiated. This practice is declining owing to a greater awareness of radiation hazards, but it is still found too often to be overlooked.

Radiation, to be sure, is still the only effective method for treating certain irritating or disfiguring skin disorders, and the patient may be the first to demand radiotherapy in full awareness of the risk involved. Radiotherapy also reduces the severe pain that accompanies ankylosing spondylitis, an arthritic disease of the spine that afflicts thousands of men and often leads to a useless or impaired life. In such cases, where irritation or pain may be severe, it is unlikely that the hazards of radiation will deter a patient from accepting radiotherapy. He will probably take the risk—especially if the risk is relatively small.*

The element of risk cannot be avoided, but the amount of risk can be reduced appreciably. X-ray equipment can be used with moderation and with good sense. Doctors should be made thoroughly aware of the hazards involved and they should be taught the most advanced

---

* In England the incidence of leukemia among men who have been treated with X radiation for ankylosing spondylitis "is about one third of one per cent; yet calculations based on the national death rates . . . show that even this low incidence is about ten times greater than would have been expected in the absence of irradiation."

methods of reducing exposure. The physician should limit the use of his equipment to those aspects of radiology with which he is thoroughly familiar. A general practitioner is not a radiologist. Where complex techniques are required to diagnose a disease or treat a patient, the patient should have the benefit of the special training and experience that come from long service in the field of radiology. There is also an area which both layman and physician can enter with equal authority—that of radiation safety. Careful shielding from scattered X rays should always be provided for sensitive areas of the body, such as the gonads, neck, and abdominal region, particularly when children and young people are being irradiated. A patient has a right to insist upon protection whenever it is feasible, and in this he has the emphatic support of the most knowledgeable authorities in the field of radiology.

The use of X-ray equipment should be carefully regulated. These devices do not belong in the hands of quacks and shoe salesmen. Technicians should be licensed personnel who have given substantial evidence of their qualifications to operate X-ray equipment. Their work requires careful training that cannot be picked up through irregular, offhand instruction. There should be compulsory periodic inspections of X-ray equipment by competent agencies. Concerted efforts must be made to bring the latest advances in radiology into physicians' offices and hospitals. Research has produced faster films, electronic devices to increase the brightness of fluoroscopic screens (with concomitant reductions in X-ray dosage), image intensifiers, and improved filters that eliminate diagnostically useless long-wave radiation. Some of these improvements are too costly for the ordinary physician; hence the need to make use of the services of a well-equipped radiologist or hospital when a program of irradiation is required. It is the responsibility of the community to see that outdated X-ray equipment is scrapped and that no one is exposed to defective and potentially harmful machines.

Unfortunately, the available evidence suggests that, in most cases, both the machines and the physicians' techniques are unsatisfactory. A recent two-year survey of diagnostic X-ray equipment in New York City, for example, showed that 92 per cent of 3,623 machines inspected by the Board of Health either were not being used properly or were defective. The survey disclosed that X-ray beams were very broad, needlessly irradiating parts of the body that were not under study. The majority of physicians who were not radiologists were unfamiliar with the safety recommendations of the National Committee on Radiation Protection. The inspectors did not find a single physician who had voluntarily followed earlier recommendations to switch from outmoded to new equipment. Although the survey covered only 35 per cent of the machines employed in the city, it included the most frequently used X-ray machines, notably those in hospitals and in the offices of radiologists.

This survey, it should be emphasized, took place in 1959 and 1960, not a half century ago, when research on radiation was still in its infancy. The survey followed a period of widespread public discussion on the hazards of radiation and nuclear fallout. It is now clear that the situation is much worse than had generally been supposed. Exposure to radiation is occurring on a scale that has no precedent in man's natural history. Millions of people in all stages of life, from the fetal to the senile, are being irradiated every year. Clearly the problem of radiation control has reached serious proportions. From the various reports "on the influence of ionizing radiation on biological systems," observes the National Advisory Committee on Radiation, ". . . it is evident that serious health problems may be created by undue exposure and that every practical means should be adopted to limit such exposure both to the individual and to the population at large."

FALLOUT

X-RAY EQUIPMENT, we noted earlier, can be turned on and off, but the radioactive wastes that enter man's environment through nuclear weapons tests and the activity of nuclear reactors are essentially beyond human control. They contaminate air, water, and food, and they irradiate everyone, irrespective of age or health. Radioactive contaminants also create problems not encountered with conventional pollutants. Ordinary contaminants usually lose their toxic properties by undergoing chemical change, but there is no loss of radioactivity involved in the chemical reactions of radio-isotopes. When radiocarbon combines with oxygen to form carbon dioxide, the carbon in the compound continues to emit beta particles. The same is true for chemical compounds formed by strontium-90. Radioactivity persists in all radio-isotopes until unstable atoms decay into stable ones.

Until recently, the layman was given a highly misleading picture of the hazards created by nuclear weapons tests. This picture was largely created by the Atomic Energy Commission, the official agency that had been made chiefly responsible for furnishing the public with information in the field of nuclear energy. For many years the A.E.C. consistently minimized the danger posed by radioactive fallout produced by nuclear weapons tests. For example, it completely ignored the extent to which food had been contaminated with strontium-90 until the problem was raised by scientists who were critical of the agency's public information policies. "In the 13th Semiannual Report of the AEC, published in 1953," notes Barry Commoner, of Washington University, "the AEC stated that the only possible hazard to humans from strontium-90 would arise from 'the ingestion of bone splinters which might be intermingled with muscle tissue during butchering and cutting of the meat.' No mention of milk was made"—or, for that matter, of vegetables and cereals. Spokesmen for the A.E.C. predicted that fallout would be uniformly distributed over the earth, so that no areas need fear concentrations of debris from nuclear weapons tests. The public was assured that the greater part of the debris sent into the stratosphere would remain aloft for a period of five to ten years. As fallout occurs very slowly, it was said, the radioactivity of short-lived radio-isotopes would be almost entirely dissipated in the stratosphere.

Actually, the radioactive debris that soars into the stratosphere stays there, on an average, less than five years. According to General Herbert B. Loper, of the Department of Defense, half the stratospheric debris produced by a nuclear explosion returns to the earth within two years. Fallout occurs three and one half times faster than Willard F. Libby, former commissioner of the A.E.C, had estimated. A model of stratospheric air circulation developed by A. W. Brewer and G. M. B. Dobson indicates that the heaviest fallout in the Northern Hemisphere occurs in the temperate zone, reaching a peak between 40 and 50 degrees north latitude—or roughly between Madrid and London in Europe and between New York City and Winnipeg in North America. Measurements made during the 1958-61 nuclear weapons test moratorium indicate that the hazard from fallout in these latitudes is substantially greater than the world-wide average.*

The rapidity with which radioactive debris descends to the earth places the danger presented by short-lived, supposedly harmless radioactive elements in a new perspective. Cesium-134 and strontium-89 have half-lives of only 2 and 56 days, respectively, but nuclear explosions produce these radioactive elements in such relatively large quantities that, if fallout is rapid, they become a serious hazard to public health. Cesium-134, like long-lived cesium-137 (another component of fallout), is an emitter of beta rays. When taken into the body, both cesium isotopes are handled metabolically like potassium; they migrate to all the soft tissues, including the reproductive organs. Strontium-89 possesses the characteristics of strontium-90; it, too, emits beta rays and tends to lodge in bone matter. Although a short-lived bone seeker like strontium-89 might seem to be relatively harmless, it should not be underestimated as a hazard to public health. "Since strontium-89 is produced more abundantly in fission than strontium-90 . . . ," the Special Subcommittee on Radiation of the Joint Committee on Atomic Energy reported in 1959, "it is possible that comparable doses to the body from the two materials could occur." The subcommittee added that "it would require 100 times

---

* Let us grant that the A.E.C. had made an honest error, but how did the agency handle the facts when it became evident from classified data that its predictions were wrong? A chronological account prepared by the Joint Committee on Atomic Energy indicates that a restudy by the A.E.C., released early in 1959, "makes no mention of [the] Defense Department study" and "maintains [the] position of a residence time of 5 to 10 years, selecting 6 years as the mean residence time of stratospheric fallout. Results of another AEC analysis, Project Ash Can, which indicated a residence time of 3 years, was discounted as being doubtful. No mention was made that the Department of Defense conclusions of residence half life of 2 years tended to support results of Project Ash Can."

more initial activity of strontium-89, whose half life is 56 days, to deliver the same dose to tissue that would be created by 1 unit of strontium-90. It is considered significant that transient levels of strontium-89 with approximately this ratio to strontium-90 have been observed in milk."

For a few weeks after a nuclear explosion, the windborne debris in the lower part of the atmosphere may contain appreciable amounts of iodine-131. Iodine-131 has a half-life of eight days. At the 1959 hearings of the Special Subcommittee on Radiation, E. B. Lewis, of the California Institute of Technology, observed that "the radioiodines in fallout are a special hazard to infants and children. This hazard arises for a variety of reasons. Radioiodine is a significant fraction of the fresh fission products released by nuclear weapons explosions. Grazing cattle ingest and inhale the radioiodines in fallout and then concentratate it in their milk. Infants and children are expected to ingest more of the isotope than will adults since fresh cow's milk is the principal source of fallout radioiodine in the human diet and young people obviously drink more fresh milk than do adults. As has long been known, iodine isotopes, natural and radioactive, concentrate in the thyroid gland. Moreover, for the same amount of radioiodine orally ingested, the infant thyroid receives some 15 to 20 times the dose that the adult thyroid receives. (Briefly, this is because more radioiodine is taken up by the infant than by the adult thyroid; as a result many more of the short-ranged iodine-131 beta rays will be generated in a gram of infant than in a gram of adult thyroid tissue.) Finally, in spite of its small size, the infant thyroid may be more susceptible than the adult thyroid to cancer induction by ionizing radiation."

No one denies that radio-isotopes produce damage when they are deposited in the human body. Controversy

tends to center around the "maximum permissible concentrations" (MPC's) that have been established for the
quantities of various radioactive elements that the human body can be allowed to accumulate.* There is nothing
safe about an MPC. An MPC constitutes the amount of
risk an official agency is prepared to inflict upon certain
individuals and the general population in carrying out
a nuclear-energy program. The U. S. Naval Radiological
Laboratory points out that any degree of exposure to
ionizing radiation produces "biological effects." "Since we
don't know that these effects can be completely recovered
from," observes the laboratory's report to the Special Subcommittee on Radiation, "we have to fall back on an
arbitrary decision about how much we will put up with;
i.e., what is 'acceptable' or 'permissible'—not a scientific
finding, but an administrative decision."

Many scientists take a grim view of the "administrative decisions" that have established the permissible
levels of strontium-90 for the general population. The
MPC for strontium-90 is measured in strontium units
(S.U.), formerly called "sunshine units." A single S.U.
is one micromicrocurie ($\mu\mu$c) of strontium-90 per gram
of calcium (a $\mu\mu$c is equal to one millionth of a millionth
of a curie; a curie essentially represents the amount of
radioactivity associated with one gram of radium). For a
number of years, the maximum permissible concentration
for strontium-90 was established by a definite although
largely unofficial procedure. The MPC originated as a
recommendation by the International Commission on
Radiological Protection (I.C.R.P.), an advisory body made

* In the United States, the term "maximum permissible concentration" is being superseded by "radiation protection guide" (RPG),
and the job of formulating "acceptable" values of exposure to
radiation has been placed in the hands of the newly formed Federal Radiation Council. These changes, however, do not affect the
substance of the discussion that follows.

up of scientists from all parts of the world. The International Commission's recommendation, in turn, was usually adopted by the National Committee on Radiation Protection (N.C.R.P.), the American affiliate of the I.C.R.P. Finally, the National Committee's recommendation was generally adopted by government agencies.

Until 1955, the recommendation of the International Commission dealt almost exclusively with problems of occupational exposure to radiation and radioactive isotopes. The problem of formulating an MPC for the general population was left in the hands of the commission's national affiliates and official agencies. This created a highly unsatisfactory situation. It made it possible for official agencies to grossly understate the hazards of nuclear weapons tests; they proceeded to evaluate all the dangers that fallout presented to the general population in terms of the large MPC established for workers in atomic plants. "The maximum permissible level of strontium-90 in the human skeleton, accepted by the International Commission on Radiological Protection, corresponds to 1000 micromicrocuries per gramme of calcium [1,000 S.U.]," noted the British Medical Research Council in the mid-1950's. "But this is the maximum permissible level for adults in special occupations and is not suitable for application to the population as a whole or to children with their greater sensitivity to radiation and greater expectation of life." To cope with this problem, the International Commission decided in 1955 that the prolonged exposure of a large population to radiation should not exceed one tenth of the maximum permissible levels adopted for occupational exposures. For all practical purposes, the commission's recommendation meant that the MPC for strontium-90 established for the general population should be reduced from 1,000 to 100 S.U.

It was not until a great deal of controversy had developed over the established MPC for strontium-90 that the National Committee, followed with undisguised reluctance by the A.E.C., adopted the "one-tenth rule" recommended by the International Commission. It soon became evident that even this 90 per cent reduction was inadequate. Finally, the International Commission made a curious, perhaps contradictory decision: It raised the MPC for workers in atomic plants from 1,000 to 2,000 S.U. but recommended that the MPC for the general population be reduced to one thirtieth of the occupational level. Thus, in a circuitous, often confusing manner, the permissible level of strontium-90 for the general population has been reduced to 67 S.U., or one fifteenth of the MPC (1,000 S.U.) that was in effect in 1954.

The problem of establishing a "suitable" MPC, however, is still unsettled. Strontium-90 is not uniformly distributed in bone matter. The element, like radium, tends to form "hot spots," some of which may exceed the average skeletal distribution many times over. To estimate the damage which skeletal concentrations of strontium-90 are likely to produce, a factor, N, should be used to increase any average result based on a uniform distribution of the element in the bone—especially in the case of adults, who form these "hot spots" more readily than children. Two Swedish investigators, A. Engström and R. Björnerstedt, who have pioneered in research on this problem, emphasize that N is not constant. The factor may vary from 6 to 60, depending upon individual metabolism and variations in the amount of strontium-90 that appear in food, air, and water. An individual who acquired an average, presumably "safe," skeletal burden of 65 S.U., for example, might well have minute "hot spots" of nearly 4,000 S.U.—enough to increase appreciably his chances of developing cancer.

"Meanwhile, what is the course of wisdom?" asks

W. O. Caster, of the University of Minnesota. "Some claim that where there is honest doubt, public safety demands that the safety standards be adjusted to cover the worst possible contingency. But if one couples Dr. Engström's estimate of 100 strontium units as the maximum permissible level for radiation workers with the International Commission's suggestion that the permissible level for a population should be one thirtieth the occupational level, it would appear that the population limit should be only three strontium units. Some children have already passed this mark. The official agencies point out that, in the absence of proof that such a level is in any way deleterious, it would be the height of irresponsibility to raise a public alarm." The proof required by official agencies, however, might not be forthcoming for ten or fifteen years.

Whatever the analytic method employed, there is no doubt that concentrations of strontium-90 in human bones have been rising steadily over the past decade. The principal source of American data on the amount of radio-strontium entering the human body is an A.E.C.-financed research project at the Lamont Geological Observatory of Columbia University under the direction of J. Laurence Kulp. Thus far, Kulp's research group has issued four reports, covering the years 1954-9. The data show that for the "Western culture" area (Europe and the United States), situated between 30 and 70 degrees north latitude, the average amount of skeletal strontium-90 in adults increased from 0.07 S.U. in 1954 to 0.31 S.U. in 1959. The amount of radio-strontium in the bones of children up to four years of age rose from 0.5 S.U. in 1955 to 2.3 S.U. in 1959, a total seven times the amount in adults. Although the body discriminates in favor of dietary calcium against strontium, the discriminatory factor varies with age. As adults no longer undergo skeletal growth, they add only about one fourth of the strontium they ingest to their bones; children, however, add about half.

The value of averaging the amount of strontium-90 in bones at a given collection point, and then averaging the averages for an entire "culture area," is highly questionable. Jack Schubert has pointed out that "when dealing with a potentially harmful agent involving the world's population, it can be misleading to use average values of strontium-90 in the bones. It is important, especially in relation to the setting of permissible levels for a world population, that we have some basis for estimating the degree to which appreciable fractions of the population accumulate two and more times the average amount." Using more suitable mathematical methods than those employed by Kulp and his colleagues, Schubert shows that 28 per cent of the skeletal specimens analyzed in the 1957-8 Kulp report "have *three* or more times the average (geometric mean) amount of strontium-90 in their bones. Over 4 per cent will have seven or more times the average! These values are appreciably greater than those of Kulp's who used incorrect averages and an incorrect distribution curve and hence underestimated the fraction of the population which would exceed the average values." *

Submerged in the avalanche of averages, estimates, and statistical extrapolations are those communities that have been heavily irradiated by fallout debris. "Substantial areas in Nevada and Utah close to the bomb testing grounds had received ten roentgens of gamma radiation as early as 1955," Caster observes. "Some 40 communities had had average doses between one and eight roentgen

---

* For the benefit of readers who are familiar with statistical methods, it might be added that a proper evaluation of Kulp's data requires a Poisson distribution, not the normal distribution employed by Kulp and his group.

units. Such doses are substantially above allowable levels for the general population—or for professional personnel for that matter." In May 1953, for example, a sudden change in weather caused the fallout "cloud" from a Nevada test series to move over well-traveled and inhabited areas near Yucca Flats. According to an account of the episode by Paul Jacobs, fairly high levels of air contamination were recorded in St. George (population, 5,000) and Hurricane (population, 1,375).* Hundreds of motor vehicles traveling the highways near the test site required decontamination, while residents of endangered communities (when they could be reached) were warned to remain indoors. At St. George, reports Jacobs, a "high degree of contamination continued for sixteen days after the shots."

Radioactive debris from the Nevada test explosions normally drifts in a northeasterly direction toward the grain and dairy states of the upper Midwest. It tends to settle out in areas where a large percentage of the American food supply is raised. As a result, high concentrations of strontium-90 have been found in food plants, especially cereals, grown in many parts of the Great Plains region. In 1957, for example, wheat samples collected from seven agricultural experiment stations in Minnesota registered concentrations of strontium-90 about 100 per cent higher than the current daily maximum permissible level (MPL) for humans over a lifetime. The largest num-

* A similar incident occurred a year later, when a large group of Marshall Islanders received high doses of radiation as a result of a hydrogen-bomb test at the A.E.C.'s Eniwetok Proving Grounds in the Pacific Ocean. Exposure to fallout was sufficiently high to induce symptoms of "radiation sickness" in many of the natives. Had the wind veered thirty miles to the south, the entire population of the islands would have been exposed to lethal doses of radiation (about 1,000 roentgens).

ber of S.U. found in one group of Minnesota samples was 200 per cent greater than the MPL.

Had a moratorium on nuclear weapons tests not been established in the autumn of 1958, the amount of strontium-90 in milk from certain collection points in the United States might well have approached or equaled the current MPL value of 33 $\mu\mu$c per liter. The A.E.C.'s "Hardtack" series of explosions in Nevada and high-yield Russian tests in Siberia, both conducted during 1958, resulted in heavy fallout. In 1959, the amount of strontium-90 in milk reached 14.6 $\mu\mu$c per liter in New York City (July 18), 18.2 in Cincinnati, Ohio (May 19), 22.6 in Spokane, Washington (May 5), and 22.8 in Atlanta, Georgia (May 5). Heavy concentrations of strontium-90 appeared in wheat and cereal products, particularly in whole-wheat bread. During February 1959, for example, the levels of strontium-90 in whole-wheat bread obtained by the A.E.C. from New York City retail markets generally exceeded the MPL value of 33 $\mu\mu$c per kilogram.*

Attempts have been made by highly responsible scientists to estimate the damage caused by the fallout debris produced to date. According to A. N. Sturtevant, professor of genetics at the California Institute of Technology, fallout will produce harmful genetic mutations

* With the resumption of nuclear weapons tests, the amount of strontium-90 in food is expected to reach unprecedented levels. It is likely that the strontium-90 in the milk supply of a number of American communities will substantially exceed the MPL of 33 $\mu\mu$c per liter. Estimates based on the Federal Radiation Council's "radiation protection guides" (RPG's) place 1962 levels of strontium-90 in milk in the lower part of "Range II" (from 20 to 200 $\mu\mu$c of strontium-90 per liter). This range requires "active surveillance and routine control" by public health authorities. It is hardly necessary to emphasize that there will be a sharp increase in skeletal burdens of strontium-90, especially in children and young adults.

in 4,000 people in the first generation and in 40,000 people in generations to come. Although these figures represent Sturtevant's latest published estimates (1959), they are calculated on the basis of the radioactive debris produced up to 1956. Since then, the total amount of fallout has increased about 70 per cent. On the basis of more up-to-date material, James Crow, president of the Genetics Society of America, estimates that 20,000 mutations will be inherited by the next generation as a result of fallout (his estimate is based on the assumption that the present world population will produce a total of two billion children). The number would reach 200,000 if nuclear testing were resumed and continued for thirty years at the 1954-8 rate.

If E. B. Lewis's "linear hypothesis" is correct, fallout may have contributed to the rising incidence of leukemia. According to Lewis's theory, the chances of acquiring leukemia increase in direct (or linear) proportion to increased irradiation. The hypothesis "predicts that constant exposure to even one sunshine unit [strontium unit] would be capable of producing about 5 to 10 cases of leukemia annually in the United States population." There seem to be very few scientists who deny that linearity exists in the middle dose range of radiation, but a great deal of controversy has arisen over Lewis's hypothesis that linearity exists at all levels of radiation, including the very low dose range involved in diagnostic X-rays and fallout. Yet there is a substantial amount of data to support his theory. Aside from the basic evidence that Lewis presented when his views were first published (1957), the linear hypothesis has gained strong support from the work of Alice Stewart and others on cancer in children (see page 170). The pelvimetries studied by Stewart and her co-workers involved dosages of only 2 to 10 rads; nevertheless, this low level of whole-body radiation directed at the fetus was enough to double its chances of acquiring cancer.

If Lewis's hypothesis is also valid for other forms of radiation-induced cancer, fallout from nuclear weapons tests may be responsible for thousands of cases of bone cancer. By using a statistical approach developed by the British Atomic Scientists Association, it is possible to make a rough but reasonable estimate of the number of such cancers that would be produced by increases in the amount of strontium-90 in human bones. A long-term average of only one strontium unit in the bones of every individual in the world may well cause 12,500 cases of bone cancer; as little as two strontium units may result in 25,000 cases. The figure increases proportionately as strontium-90 becomes part of the human skeleton. It is sobering to note that if the world population were to acquire an average skeletal concentration of 20 strontium units—or one third of the current maximum permissible concentration—a quarter of a million people might be afflicted with bone cancer.

All of these estimates and hypotheses may be wrong, but thus far there are no convincing reasons for believing that they err on the side of pessimism. "The by-products of atomic fission are highly destructive to protoplasm," observe Ralph and Mildred Buchsbaum, "and in unique ways which present problems that were never posed by the other hazards man has introduced into his environment by his technology. The dangers are at present underestimated, rather than exaggerated, in the opinion of most biologists."

THE NUCLEAR AGE

IF NUCLEAR WEAPONS TESTS were ended permanently, we would still be confronted with far-reaching dangers created by the peacetime uses of nuclear energy. In contrast to the minuscule quantity of radioactive substances to which man had access before 1940, the nuclear-energy industry produces millions of curies of waste materials every year. The "high-level" wastes created by the reprocessing of partially spent nuclear fuels may contain as much as several thousand curies of radioactive substances per gallon. More than 65 million gallons of these lethal materials are stored in giant underground tanks at three locations in the United States. So-called "intermediate" and "low-level" wastes are discharged directly into the ground. Radioactive substances in liquid form, for example, are piped into gravel-filled trenches and allowed to percolate into the soil. Over 2½ million curies of solid and liquid waste products have been disposed of in the ground. The liquid wastes "work their way slowly into ground water," observes the A.E.C. in its 1959 *Annual Report,* "leaving all or part of their radioactivity held either chemically or physically in the soil." To put the key thought in this statement less obliquely: Part of the radioactivity reaches the ground water and passes into man's environment.

Large quantities of "low-level" wastes have been discharged into rivers. At Hanford, Washington, for example, about 2,000 curies of substances that have been made radioactive by neutrons in reactors are released daily into the Columbia River. After making a survey of the Priest Rapids–Paterson section of the river, a group of U. S. Public Health Service investigators pointed out that "values as high as 2.2×10^{-3} $\mu c/gm$. [.002 micro-curies per gram] have been found in the muscle of white fish near Priest Rapids." The writers reported that other river organisms "had gross beta activity densities considerably higher than adult fish, but these organisms are not utilized to any extent by humans. Thus, their major significance is in transmitting this activity to other organisms in the food chain. Fish as well as ducks, geese and other animals, may consume these organisms." These higher animals, it should be noted, are consumed by man.

In addition to using rivers as a means of disposal, the A.E.C. has dumped 65,000 concrete-lined drums containing "low-level" radioactive garbage into the Atlantic and Pacific oceans. Owing to the corrosive action of sea water, the porosity of the concrete liners, and the high water pressures at the floor of the ocean, the drums may last as little as ten years. Approximately 60,000 curies of radioactivity were disposed of in the oceans before the A.E.C., yielding to widespread public protest, declared a "moratorium" on this type of disposal in all Atlantic and many Pacific coastal waters pending a further study of how effectively the wastes are retained by their containers. The A.E.C., however, is by no means the worst contributor to radioactive pollution of the oceans. British authorities allow their Windscale installations to pump as much as 10,000 curies of short-lived radio-isotopes into the Irish Sea every month.

What happens to these wastes when they enter the environment of fresh- and salt-water marine life? Generally, ecological factors play a number of ugly tricks on man; it has been clearly established that radioactive materials in water tend to be concentrated by plankton, algae, mollusks, and fish. "Available substances are rapidly taken up by the biota, never remaining long in the water to be diluted and washed away," observes Lauren

R. Donaldson, of the University of Washington. "This is dramatically demonstrated following an atomic test in which radioactive materials are deposited in the water. Within hours, the great bulk of these materials is to be found in the living organisms. Plankton and some of the algae, which are the key organisms in the food chain, may concentrate within themselves more than a thousand times the amount of radioactive substances found in the sea water. The herbivorous fish and invertebrates have lower concentrations of radionuclides at any given time than do the plants on which they feed, and progressing along the food chain to the carnivores the concentrations become lower and lower."

There have been cases, however, in which the concentration of radioactive elements was higher in fish and mollusks than in plants. In a study of fallout on a four-acre pond near Cincinnati, L. R. Setter and A. S. Goldin, of the U. S. Public Health Service, found extreme variations in the concentration of radioactive isotopes among different species of water life. In some algae the amount of radioactivity was only 20 times greater than that in the water, but bass had from 300 to 400 times more, and snails from 1,000 to 3,000. Data supplied by Richard F. Foster, of the Hanford Laboratories, indicate that whereas algae in the Columbia River concentrate radiocesium by a factor of 1,000 to 5,000, fish concentrate the element by a factor of 5,000 to 10,000.* In any case, as one organism is nourished by another, the radio-isotopes reappear to a greater or lesser degree in the bodies of higher species. The route may be direct and simple or

---

* Foster's report, incidentally, shows that algae can concentrate radio-potassium in amounts as much as a million times greater than that in river water, and fish can concentrate strontium-90 as much as a thousand times.

long and complex, but eventually a portion of the radioactive garbage finds its way back to man.

It is rather alarming to speculate on the direction the nuclear age may yet take. According to the Committee on the Effects of Atomic Radiation on Oceanography and Fisheries of the National Academy of Sciences, "300 nuclear powered ships of all nations will be in service by 1975. These ships could then potentially release to the marine environment approximately 5000 curies per year from expansion water, some 3400 curies per year from leakage, and some 9×10^5 [900,000] curies per year from the ion exchange beds." The total: 908,400 curies per year. At the same time, new reactors on the land can be expected to create ever-mounting problems of waste disposal. It has been estimated that if nuclear power furnished 10 per cent of America's current electrical output (a distinct possibility in the next few decades), there would exist in the world about 150 billion curies of radioactive isotopes from this source alone, including 2.6 billion curies of strontium-90 and 2.3 billion curies of cesium-137. These figures, let it be noted, do not include radioactive wastes that would be produced by nuclear power plants in other countries. Methods for the permanent disposal of such highly lethal materials would have to be "foolproof." If any miscalculations were made and the wastes began to seep uncontrollably into man's environment, they would cause a staggering amount of damage.

The nuclear age could have profound and far-reaching effects upon existing ecological patterns. Until recently, biologists assumed that the sensitivity of living things to radiation increases with the level of their evolutionary complexity. For example, viruses absorb between 50,000 and 100,000 roentgens before half or more of their number are killed; spore-forming bacteria, between 20,000 and 50,000; the weevil, between 1,000 and 2,000 roentgens. But mammals such as the dog, the goat, and man begin to succumb to whole-body doses of less than 500 roentgens. In reviewing the striking differences in radio-resistance between lower and higher forms of life, many biologists concluded that if man and other mammals could be protected from radiation, the rest of the biosphere would more or less take care of itself.

It seems unlikely, however, that this conclusion is correct. There appear to be critical periods in the development of many highly radio-resistant species during which they can be damaged or killed by fairly low levels of radiation. For example, it requires only 160 roentgens to kill half the eggs of the fruit fly during the early stages of cell division, whereas 100,000 roentgens are needed to achieve the same result with adults. The organism is 600 times more radio-resistant at one stage of its development than at another. As plants and lower animals tend to concentrate relatively large quantities of radioactive isotopes in their cells, a level of environmental contamination "harmless" to man may prove to be very harmful to less-developed species. The use of the soil, atmosphere, and bodies of water as dumping grounds for nuclear wastes could result in serious ecological imbalances that would eventually affect man. "When radioactive isotopes are released into the environment," observes K. Z. Morgan, of the Oak Ridge Laboratory, "they usually enter into complex physical and biological cycles and into food chains and may exhibit unexpected movements or concentrations. It is through such mechanisms that dangerous long-lived radionuclides such as strontium-90 and cesium-137 are able to enter our food sources. These ecological food chains are actually circular in nature or web-like and have a limited number of links. Serious consequences would follow if too many of these food links were broken."

Morgan emphasizes that the damage can be very subtle. Radiation may reduce the mobility of an animal or impair its sensory organs, such as the eyes. It may reduce the organism's fertility. "Also, if a small dose has any effect at all at any stage in the life cycle of an organism, then chronic radiation at this level can be more damaging than a single massive dose which comes at a time when only resistant stages are present. Finally stress and changes in mutation rates may be produced even when there is no immediately obvious effect on survival of irradiated individuals."

Nuclear energy is associated with such huge problems in human affairs that the subtle dangers it creates for the biosphere may seem to be negligible. The tendency to deal with the atom in terms of massive destruction and large-scale economic exploitation may lower our guard and lead to serious ecological disturbances. Although the wastes discharged into the environment contain, for the most part, short-lived radio-isotopes, the daily volume of effluent is immense and the flow continuous. The radio-isotopes are picked up, concentrated, and circulated in increasing amounts by key organisms in the vicinity of nuclear reactors and processing establishments until many plants and animals become heavily contaminated. The smaller number of long-lived radio-isotopes are carried further into major food chains that involve millions of people. Before creating new centers of radioactivity and adding to existing problems of waste disposal, we would do wisely to ask whether all the hazards of exposure to low-level radiation have been explored and whether all the alternatives to nuclear power have been exhausted. "It is not too late at this point for us to reconsider old decisions and make new ones," observes Walter Schneir in an excellent article on radioactive wastes. "For the moment at least, a choice is available."

CHAPTER SEVEN

Human Ecology

SURVIVAL AND HEALTH

DESPITE mounting problems and difficulties, most official statements on environmental change tend to be reassuring and optimistic. We are told repeatedly, for example, that the amount of strontium-90 in a quart of milk or the quantity of DDT in a fruit is "trivial"; that in order to ingest harmful doses of a radioactive element or a pesticide residue, an individual would have to consume enormous quantities of a contaminated food at a single sitting. These piecemeal explanations are little more than subterfuges. Many toxicants appear in all the fruits and vegetables we consume; in fact, strontium-90 and DDT are in almost every food in the modern diet. We ingest these substances daily with nearly every glass and spoon we raise to our lips. They appear in the air we breathe and the water we drink. Since the 1940's, strontium-90 and DDT have become an integral part of man's environment; the toxicants are almost as widespread as bacteria and dust particles.

An over-all view of our synthetic environment, even if cursory and superficial, reveals a picture worse than that disclosed by the most exhaustive specialized investigations. Foods are sprayed not only with DDT but with a large assortment of inorganic and organic insecticides; they contain not only strontium-90 but additional radioisotopes created by man. A large part of the modern diet consists of highly processed foods to which questionable artificial materials have been added. Although the average man is engaging in less and less physical activity, his intake of carbohydrates and fats is very high. The growth of urban centers has been accompanied by increasing air and water pollution. The anxieties and tensions of modern life promote the consumption of cigarettes, drugs, and analgesics. Modern man ingests an appalling variety of toxic materials every day, many of which are additive or interact in the body to produce a synergistic effect.* The initial damage created by these toxicants is likely to be disregarded, partly because the more immediate symptoms of low-level, chronic poisoning, such as persistent fatigue and a continual sense of ill-being, are so common that they are no longer taken seriously.

How does this conclusion compare with evidence that human longevity has been increasing? Actually, the

* Two widely used organophosphorus insecticides, EPN and malathion, for example, are known synergists; each is toxic when ingested singly, but when they are taken together, EPN inhibits the hydrolyzing enzyme that detoxifies malathion, thus producing a toxic effect that is more than additive. Ionizing radiation, to cite another example, is not only carcinogenic in its own right, but also reinforces the activity of chemical carcinogens in tobacco smoke. As John W. Berg, associate editor of *Cancer*, notes: ". . . what we gain with cigarette filters we probably lose to fallout from atomic explosions."

claim that man is living longer today than he did a half century ago requires qualification. "It is important to realize that most of the gains in longevity have come about through prevention of mortality at young ages," observes James M. Hundley, of the National Institute of Health. "Great progress has been made in this sector. Relatively little has been gained in older age groups." Since 1900 about 19 years have been added to the life expectancy of newly born white male children. A white male born at the turn of the century had a life expectancy at birth of 48.2 years; by 1958, newly born white males had a life expectancy of 67.2 years. But the gain diminishes sharply after the second decade of life and virtually disappears after the sixth. A man who is 20 years of age can expect to live 7.8 years longer than his counterpart in 1900; a man of 45 years of age, only 2.9 years; a man 65 years of age, merely 1.2 years. A child today has a better chance of reaching the age of 40, but after that his life expectancy is not appreciably greater than what it would have been at the turn of the century.

Moreover, it should not be forgotten that in 1900 millions of Americans lived in an environment in which survival was almost miraculous by present-day standards. The majority of urban dwellers lived in slums with a minimum of sanitation and medical care. A large number of children worked in factories. Their parents were shackled to a grim industrial routine for ten or twelve hours a day in patently unhealthful surroundings. Almost any improvement in social conditions or medical techniques would have rescued large numbers of people from premature death and added substantially to their life span. Today, sanitation, housing, working conditions, and income have been improved greatly, while medicine has scaled undreamed-of heights. Nevertheless, most of the increase in longevity is due to the fact that more children survive the diseases of infancy and adolescence today than two generations ago. What this means, in effect, is that if it weren't for the extraordinary medical advances and great improvements in the material conditions of life, today's adult might well have a much shorter life span than his grandparents had. This is a remarkable indication of failure. It suggests that modern man would find it very difficult to survive outside a medical and pharmaceutical hothouse.

What does life in a medical and pharmaceutical hothouse entail? The answer, in cold statistics, is shocking. Nearly 41 per cent of the American people have some form of chronic illness.* Many of these individuals are confined to wheel chairs, nursing homes, and hospital beds, faced with lifelong pain and inactivity. The statistics include numerous victims of heart disease, whose existence is marred by continual apprehension and fear. They include hundreds of thousands of cancer victims, a large percentage all but departed from the pale of the living. Worse still, however, the likelihood exists that the hothouse will begin to fall apart as the pace of chemicalization, urbanization, and pollution is increased. We have yet to feel the full burden of disease slowly being created by nuclear weapons tests, motorcar exhausts, and the newer chemical additives in our food.

We are exchanging health for mere survival. We have begun to measure man's biological achievements, not in terms of his ability to live a vigorous, physically untroubled life, but in terms of his ability to preserve his

---

* "About 40.9 per cent of persons living in the United States were reported to have one or more chronic conditions," reports the U. S. Public Health Service. "While some of these conditions were relatively minor, others were serious conditions such as heart disease, diabetes, or mental illness." Ten per cent of the American population are forced to limit their activity because of chronic conditions.

mere existence in an increasingly distorted environment.
Today, survival often entails ill health and rapid physical
degeneration. We are prepared to accept the fact that a
relatively young individual will suffer from frequent
headaches and digestive disturbances, continual nervous
tension, insomnia, a persistent "cigarette cough," a mouth-
ful of decaying teeth, and respiratory ailments every
winter. We expect his physique to acquire the rotundity
of a barrel shortly after the onset of middle age; we find
nothing extraordinary in the fact that he is incapable of
running more than a few yards without suffering loss
of breath or walking a few miles without suffering exhaustion.

What, then, is health? At the very least, health must
be regarded as the absence of all the persistant pains,
aches, tensions, and physical disturbances now accepted
as a "normal" part of life. A healthy body is not a burden;
it does not provoke an irritating awareness of its presence without reason. When we are in good health, we
sense that our bodies are completely at our command,
that they are in the service of our purposes and desires.
Normally the "sound body lives in silence," observes Alexis
Carrel. "We do not hear, we do not feel, its working. The
rhythms of our existence are expressed by cenesthesic
impressions which, like the soft whirring of a sixteen-
cylinder motor, fill the depths of our consciousness when
we are in silence and meditation. The harmony of organic functions gives us a feeling of peace."

This is, of course, a minimum definition of health—
a definition that might be taken for granted if it were
not for the fact that, as Carrel adds, many people, "although they are not ill, are not in good health. Perhaps
the quality of some of their tissues is defective. The secretions of such gland, or such mucosa, may be insufficient
or too abundant. The excitability of their nervous system,

exaggerated. Their organic functions, not exactly correlated in space or in time. Or their tissues, not as capable of resisting infections as they should be." Carrel is obviously concerned with complex, interacting biochemical factors that are often difficult to pinpoint and measure in the laboratory. Nevertheless, many individuals whose response to conventional diagnostic tests indicates that they are "normal" and hence "healthy" undoubtedly lack the energy, recuperative powers, and "harmony of organic functions" required for the full enjoyment of life. Although these individuals are considered "healthy" by current medical standards, they are not getting what they should out of life. In many cases, they can be expected to succumb prematurely to chronic diseases.

It is difficult to formulate a complete definition of health in general terms. Today, "glowing health," to use an old phrase, is very uncommon among adults. As a result, we are usually constrained to think of it not as the attribute of a population but rather as that of a few individuals. We have not yet determined the potentialities of physical development for the community as a whole. Anthropologists and physicians have explored the relics of the past and traveled to remote primitive areas in an attempt to find evidence of robust, healthy communities. These explorations have yielded a great deal of useful information, but very few of the reports give us an adequate idea of what health *could* be if science and technology were placed completely in the service of human needs. Man is capable of being a great deal more than he is today—physically as well as intellectually—if his resources are employed in a rational manner.

The term "rational" should not be taken to mean natural or primitive. Man could not have advanced beyond a level of precarious subsistence if he had not consciously altered his natural environment and hammered it into a form that favored human life. The change was made at the expense of other species and, to some extent, by violating time-honored ecological relationships. Civilization was achieved by clearing forests, draining swamps, restricting animal predators, replacing many wild botanical species with food plants, fertilizing the soil, cultivating crops, probing the earth for fuels and metals—in short, by rearranging the natural world to satisfy human needs for food, shelter, and leisure. Modern man now has the power, knowledge, and resources to do substantially better than both his ancestors and his primitive contemporaries. His technology and science have given him an enormous influence over many natural forces. Chemistry has illuminated part of the darkness that once surrounded important aspects of soil development, nutrition, and physiology. In conjunction with research in microbiology and physiology, it has given society powerful therapeutic agents, such as antibiotics and hormones. Technology can remove much of the drudgery that burdens human life and leave men free to use their bodies and minds for highly satisfying activities. Work can be pleasant as well as useful. Neither science nor technology, however, is a substitute for a balanced relationship between man and nature. Medicine and machinery may modify this relationship, but they cannot replace it. Few drugs are as effective as biological resistance to disease; no system of technology is likely to free man from his dependence on soil, plants, and animals. The two spheres, natural and synthetic, must be brought into a complementary relationship based on a clear understanding of man's needs as an animal organism and the effects of his behavior on the natural world.

A study of the interaction between man and nature may be called human ecology. Our synthetic environment is the product of man's interaction with the natural world, just as a dam is the product of a beaver's interaction with a stream and forest. The improverishment and destruction of the soil, repeated insect infestations, and the rising incidence of certain diseases represent the reaction of the natural world to man's adverse environmental changes. To become what biologists term a "dominant organism," man is compelled to make sweeping demands upon nature, but nature, in turn, makes demands that man must fulfill if he is to enjoy health and well-being. Whether he likes it or not, there are "rules of the game," which must be obeyed if an environmental change is to advance human vigor, resistance to disease, and longevity. When these rules, simple as they may be, are transgressed, nature takes its revenge in the form of ill health and disease. When they are obeyed, man's life can be full, creative, and remarkably free of physical impairment.

ECOLOGY AND HEALTH

IN A WITTY REVIEW of popular attitudes toward food, David Cort remarks that he has encountered absurdly conflicting dietary recommendations in books and articles on nutrition. One authority advises his readers to avoid fat; another advises that it should be eaten, on the theory that fat is the least fattening of all foods. Potatoes have been alternately damned and praised; mixed meals have been both frowned upon and approved; the consumption of alcohol, criticized and recommended. "The cruelty and irresponsibility of offering one single, standard dietary solution for everybody is obvious," Cort adds. "What a person eats is, in many important respects, his life. But every individual is different from every other individual. No doctrinaire solution will work for them all. Each individual has conditioned habits of eating, of taste, of appetite, of expenditure of energy, of nervous rhythms and, most important of all, of metabolism. Few modern doctors have the interest, time or genius to find out all about any one individual; and many are themselves overweight. But the individual has the time and interest and, at least about himself, perhaps the genius. After all, it's his life."

Although Cort's remarks are confined to nutrition, they are quite relevant to a number of problems in human ecology. It would be an error to form rigid concepts of a normal man, a normal diet, or a normal way of life. Any such image would be woefully lacking in biochemical and physiological support. The biologist and physician must still admit, as Carrel did nearly a quarter of a century ago, that "most of the questions put to themselves by those who study human beings remain without answer. Immense regions of our inner world are still unknown." Impressive advances, to be sure, have been made during the past two decades in solving major problems of cellular biochemistry, endocrinology, and physiology. Knowledge of the transformation of energy in the cell is very far advanced, for example, and great strides have been made in understanding the chemistry of the genetic material in the cell's nucleus. Despite this newly acquired knowledge, however, nutritionists have an extremely limited understanding of the function of many trace elements in the body and of the way in which vitamins prevent deficiency diseases. The nutritional requirements of the various tissues, essential details of the blood-forming system, the mechanisms of resistance to disease, and many key relationships within the body await clearer understanding.

The human organism is extremely sensitive to very small quantities of hormones and nutrients. A variation by only a few drops in the daily output of insulin, a pancreatic hormone, will determine whether an individual will handle sugar properly or succumb to diabetes. A difference of a few thousandths of a gram (milligrams) in the intake of certain vitamins and trace elements makes for either well-being or nutritional disorders. According to the National Research Council, a man twentyfive years of age requires a daily intake of 1.6 milligrams of thiamine and riboflavin, 7.5 milligrams of vitamin C, and 12 milligrams of iron to preserve good health. His minimum daily requirements of iodine and copper are believed to be as little as 0.1 and 0.2 milligrams, respectively. If the daily intake of these nutrients is reduced by a few thousandths of a gram or less for a long period of time, the result will be a marked impairment of health. Despite the minute quantities involved, deficiencies of vitamins and minerals occur on a fairly large scale in the United States. If A. F. Morgan and L. M. Odland are correct in their claim that a dry, roughened skin and lesions of the eyes and mouth "may be considered a useful pointer to possible dietary faults," about 50 per cent of the adolescents examined in the affluent northeastern states and 20 per cent in the western states may have nutritional disorders.

We tend to look upon diseases as though they were localized disturbances, confined to definite parts of the body. Although it is customary to acknowledge the body's unity in sickness and in health, the whole is often overlooked in favor of the parts, and vital interrelationships are ignored in favor of isolated events. Actually, every major deficiency and physical impairment has far-reaching effects. "Disease consists of a functional and structural disorder," Carrel notes. "Its aspects are as numerous as our organic activities. There are diseases of the stomach, of the heart, of the nervous system, etc. But in illness the body preserves the same unity as in health. It is sick as a whole. No disturbance remains strictly confined to a single organ. Physicians have been led to consider each disease as a specialty by the old anatomical conception of the human being. Only those who know man both in his parts and in his entirety, simultaneously under his anatomical, physiological, and mental aspects, are capable of understanding him when he is sick."

A clear understanding of illness and health requires a greater appreciation not only of man but of men. Physical needs and responses vary enormously from one individual to another. Roger J. Williams, one of America's most eminent biochemists, emphasizes that within the same racial groups, even in the same families, men differ from one another in the shape and weight of their vital organs, the composition of body fluids, the output of endocrine glands, the rate of metabolism, temperature control, and many other respects. Individual differences in the amount of nutrients required for health and in the amount of nutrients absorbed by the body are of major practical importance. Individual requirements of calcium, trace elements, amino acids, and vitamins are highly variable. For example, two normal five-year-old children who ate the same food and were exposed to the same environmental conditions showed a great variation in the amount of calcium they retained from their diets. One child retained 264 milligrams of calcium per day for 45 days, whereas the other retained 469 milligrams, a difference of nearly 80 per cent. A high degree of variability is also found in individual responses to common environmental toxicants. Williams cites an account of 78 men who were exposed to vapors of carbon tetrachloride, of whom 15 suffered acute poisoning. Six became sufficiently ill to require hospitalization. "All were white men within 5 to 8 years of the same age and in general good

health . . . ," observes Fredrich H. Harris, the source for
Williams's account. "All 15 of the men poisoned were exposed from 3 to 8 hours; however, many of those who
developed no symptoms were exposed for a similar length
of time or longer."

The fact that man's knowledge of important bodily
processes is incomplete and that many individuals exhibit
marked deviations from "normal" responses and needs
does not imply that the role of medicine is inconsequential
in promoting health or that scientific generalizations are
useless. The healthiest of men will undoubtedly require
medical attention at some time in their lives, and every
physician must use physiological and anatomical generalizations as points of departure for the diagnosis of a
disorder. Basic research in biochemistry and physiology
promises to increase vastly our understanding of the preconditions for human health and well-being. But a phenomenon does not cease to exist because it cannot be
readily explained by current methods and theories. On the
contrary, we are often profoundly affected by phenomena
that are too complex to lend themselves to precise analysis
at the present stage of scientific development. The way
in which stress produces illness and the role that nutrition
plays in the occurrence and prevention of chronic diseases
constitute fields of research that have scarcely been penetrated. It would be a major setback if the roles of these
factors were minimized simply because they present
formidable problems to research. Man must try to conserve many practices that, on the basis of long experience,
are known to promote good health, even if the reasons why
they are beneficial cannot be stated in precise biochemical
terms.

What are some of these practices? As it is clear that
our bodily functions are interdependent, we should not
permit any part of our biological equipment to atrophy.

This means that we must use all the parts of our bodies. Our musculature must be as fully employed as our minds. Many activities and experiences that have been restricted by our sheltered civilization seem to play important roles in preserving health. There is a suspicion that modern man indirectly harms his body by failing to use certain physiological resources that once supported his ancestors during periods of hunger and cold. "There exists in the body of man, as of all animals, biological mechanisms for the storage of food developed for meeting the irregularities and cyclical changes in nature," Rene Dubos writes. "It may still turn out that a nutritional way of living permitting continuous growth at a maximum rate may have unfortunate distant results. Fasting fads may have some justification after all by providing an opportunity for the operation of certain emergency mechanisms built by nature into the human body."

Although it remains to be seen whether this conclusion will be accepted by nutritionists and physicians, it is reasonably clear that a one-sided manner of life is biologically undesirable. An existence anchored in either muscular exertion or inactivity, surfeit or poverty, stress or an overly sheltered manner of life, tends to produce physiological disequilibrium. A prolonged period of muscular exertion causes marked damage, whereas protracted physical inactivity appears to increase both the effect and the incidence of heart and circulatory disorders. When the coronary arteries of dogs are surgically narrowed to simulate atherosclerosis, a lack of exercise makes it difficult for new blood vessels to form and provide more blood to nourish the diseased area of the heart muscle. There also seems to be more coronary illness among men whose occupations are sedentary than among those who engage in physical work. In contrast to the well-exercised individual, the "physically inactive individual shows signs of aging earlier in life," emphasizes Hans Kraus, of New York University. "He exists physiologically at a lower potential and is less well-equipped to maintain homeostasis [stable bodily conditions] and to meet daily stresses. This low level of function, combined with enforced suppression of the 'fight and flight' response, enhances the incidence of disease."

Not only does health require all the elements of a full life; it also requires that they exist in balance. A moderate amount of exertion, a balanced intake of nutriment, and a reasonable amount of exposure to stress are necessary for the maintenance of well-being. Almost any kind of excess is harmful. This has become apparent in respect to nutrition. "In laboratory experiments rats fed an unlimited diet were found to die sooner than animals prevented from gaining weight by a diet severely restricted in quantity but well balanced in composition," Dubos observes. "Likewise insurance statisticians have repeatedly emphasized that in man the obese have a short expectancy of life. Indeed, obesity is now publicized as the most common nutritional disease of Western society. This was apparently true also in Imperial Rome, as during all periods of great material prosperity.* 'In the old days,' wrote Lucretius in the fifth book of *De Rerum Natura*, 'lack of food gave languishing limbs to Lethe; contrariwise today surfeit of things stifles us.' Thus, history repeats itself. Like the prosperous Romans of two thousand years ago, countless men of the Western world today are digging their own graves through over-eating."

Finally, if man is to maintain good health, he requires diversity. It is hardly necessary to emphasize that

* And in periods of social decline and demoralization as well. The pursuit of "pleasure," which affluent Romans of the Imperial Age carried to the point of license, would have been frowned upon during the Periclean Age, when ancient Athens, too, enjoyed "great material prosperity."

a healthy psyche and a rounded response to stress are nourished by a variety of experiences and by diversified surroundings. However, it does need to be emphasized that variety is also necessary for the satisfaction of man's nutritional needs. By limiting his selection of foods, he may fail to acquire nutrients known to exist in natural foods but not yet identified by chemists or nutritionists. "Because we know that unidentified factors exist in foods of plant and animal origin," observes George M. Briggs, of the National Institutes of Health, "it is wisest to eat a wide variety of foods from the many excellent food groups . . ." If this is done regularly, Briggs emphasizes, it is unnecessary to supplement the diet with vitamins and so-called health foods. It might be added that if food such as grain were not overly processed, it would be unnecessary to "enrich" bread with synthetic vitamins, which replace only part of the valuable nutrients lost in the milling process. In general, the more a food is processed, the greater the likelihood that identified nutrients as well as unidentified ones will be removed.

Completeness, balance, and diversity should be regarded as practical ecological concepts—as important in producing healthy human communities as they are in producing stable plant-animal communities. Indeed, it is not farfetched to say that when these concepts are correctly applied, they promote human health because they produce a stable ecosystem of men, animals, and plants. In the last analysis, the ecology of health is grounded in natural ecology. A complete way of life for man presupposes unrestricted access to the countryside as well as the town, to soil as well as to pavement, to flora and fauna as well as to libraries and theaters. A balanced way of life presupposes a lasting equilibrium between land and city; animals, men, and plants; air, water, and industry. Diversity presupposes an awareness that nearly every species perpetuates the stability of the biosphere, either directly or indirectly. As the city encroaches on the land, however, human life becomes increasingly restricted to a polluted, nerve-racking urban environment. As the city begins to dominate the land, physical activity yields to sedentary forms of work. Finally, as the aggregations of population swell to massive proportions, foods become laden with chemicals and human activities are standardized. By oversimplifying the natural environment, we have created an incomplete man who lives an unbalanced life in a standardized world. Such a man is ill—not only morally and psychologically, but physically.

ECOLOGY IN USE

OUR ENVIRONMENT DIFFICULTIES would be understandable if we knew nothing about the requirements for a balanced relationship between man and nature. We could then answer every reproach with a confession of ignorance. Today, however, we know too much about ecology to have any excuse whatsoever for many of the abuses that are perpetrated in agriculture, food production, and urban life. The time is approaching when the *ad hoc* measures with which we have tried to stave off the problems of environmental change will have to be supplanted by lasting ecological solutions.

Ecology, as has been noted in an earlier chapter, deals with the interrelationships of living things (including man) and their environment. The more these interrelationships are explored, the more evident become the interdependence of most organisms in a given locality and the needs that each species fulfills for the others.

Most ecological studies are limited and highly concrete, but the material at hand suggests a number of practical generalizations that are relevant to the problems discussed thus far, particularly those of agriculture and land use.

A rational agricultural program must begin by taking into account the natural characteristics of the soil. "Soil productivity is not simply a matter of available chemicals," observes Edward Higbee, of Clark University. "It is also heavily dependent upon good structure, aggregation, texture, mellowness, and microorganic life." Many of these characteristics are predetermined by the natural history of a given area, including its ecology under virgin conditions, its underlying rock formation, and its prevailing climate. In addition, there are likely to be important differences in the soils of individual farms owing to variations in the slope of the land, in drainage conditions, and in the depth of the solum, or true soil, in relation to underlying layers of clay and rock. The configuration of the land determines, to a large extent, the optimal conditions of growth for different kinds of vegetation, especially in rolling or hilly country. Some areas will be best suited for pasture, others for field crops. On many farms in eastern sections of the United States, a sizable acreage of land should almost certainly be returned to timber. Attempts to exploit these soils for the cultivation of food and grazing often result in extensive erosion and unsatisfactory crops.

If no attempts were made to modify a natural ecological pattern, agriculture would be impossible, and, in many cases, superbly improved crop lands would be reclaimed by the forest and irrigated soils would again become unproductive. But we cannot ignore the ecological factors that clearly limit the cultivation of many foods. Large areas of land are now supporting crops for which they are definitely not suited, and society would profit more by giving a freer rein to nature than by forcing the soil to produce a low quality of vegetation. The dry plains from the Dakotas to western Texas, for example, were meant to be range lands, not crop lands. Weather conditions are too uncertain for the cultivation of grain, and the area suffers from repeated sieges of drought, whose effects are only aggravated by the systematic cultivation of food. The productivity of the arid plains is notoriously low, and attempts to grow commercial crops have resulted in widespread deterioration of the soil.

In most cases, the best soils of the world were developed under highly varied forms of vegetation. Although certain plant groups seemed to dominate the landscape of particular regions, a closer view usually disclosed a great diversity of species. The uniformity of the American prairies, long regarded as a "desert of grass," was an illusion. "Many virgin forests cannot display so great a variety of plant and animal life as the now nearly vanished native grasslands . . . ," Higbee writes. "For the patient individual who walks slowly and watches closely it is a world of infinite variety in small forms and subtle colors." Although agriculture can never completely restore this variety, it can try to approximate it, not only to please the eye but to create a more complex ecological pattern for purposes of controlling pests and conserving the soil. Indeed, it would be wise to diversify as well as to rotate crops. Certainly no moderate-sized farm on forest soils should be without timber, and even on the prairies it is no longer necessary to prove to the farmer that he has much to gain by planting trees as shelter belts against the wind and as oases for bird life.

To achieve a lasting, stable agriculture, we must reserve a place for livestock on the modern farm. Not only are meat and dairy cattle sources of manure, but their mere presence tends to restrain the exploitation of crop lands. Most farmers who own herds of cattle are obliged, in order to feed the animals, to cultivate soil-protecting legumes; willingly or not, they thus follow practices that conserve the land. On the whole, however, the trend has been away from mixed forms of agriculture, in which both food plants and livestock are raised on the same agricultural unit. The small farmer, faced with heavy competition from larger enterprises, has begun to specialize; he either raises livestock or cultivates a limited number of commercial crops. Dairying, one of the most important forms of mixed agriculture, is more or less on the decline throughout the United States, except in parts of the South. The number of cows and heifers kept for milk has dropped more than 20 per cent since 1945.

It need not be emphasized that the oversimplification of agriculture creates ideal conditions for the invasion and proliferation of pests. But even variety in plant life and the presence of livestock are not likely to be effective in helping to control pests if the land is being exploited. Ecologists have found that an overgrazed range, for example, tends to attract a large number of rodents and insects. "It is generally observed . . . that jack rabbits are usually most numerous where the range is poorest and the grass most sparse," notes Edward H. Graham, of the U. S. Soil Conservation Service. In a discussion on insect pests, Graham adds: "Even the abundance of grasshoppers, so destructive of crops and range vegetation, can be related in some degree to intensity of land use. Weese . . . has been credited with the statement that a barbed wire fence is the best device for controlling range insects, meaning that controlled grazing which permits good grass will automatically reduce the number of injurious insect forms."

The effective control of pests requires an appreciation of many complex factors, some of which may seem far removed from the outbreak of an infestation but play an important role in its occurrence. Albrecht has placed a great deal of emphasis on the role of soil fertility in building up the resistance of plants to insect predators. Research at the University of Missouri suggests that certain species of insects are attracted to crops grown on deficient soils. As soil fertility is improved, the infestation declines. Each host plant and each insect species, of course, constitutes a separate problem that can be solved only on its own terms. Unwise methods of fertilizing the soil may actually make it easier for an infestation to occur. For example, if nitrogen fertilizer is used excessively, it produces heavy vegetative growth, but the maturity of the plant is delayed and its cell walls are thin and are easily penetrated by disease-causing organisms. These lush, immature plants, low in resistance to pathogens, tend to attract insect predators and often pave the way for a serious infestation.

One of the most harmful misconceptions in agriculture is that all predators of crops are exclusively injurious and should be completely destroyed. Mention has been made of the valuable role played by forest rodents in limiting insect infestations (see pages 56-7); similar evidence can be adduced from areas such as the plains, where rodents have been singled out for vigorous extermination campaigns. In a study of the high plains grasshopper, Claude Wakeland observes that in some areas, rats, mice, and gophers "have devoured a great many grasshopper eggs, nymphs, and adults. Doubtless they have destroyed various forms of the species far more extensively than the meagre data available indicates." On the plains, rodents have become pests as a result of overgrazed ranges and the extermination campaigns conducted against the coyote, which feeds primarily on carrion and small mammals. Ecological studies show that 20 per cent or more of the coyote's diet consists of insects; during periods of heavy infestations, it feeds almost exclusively on grasshoppers. To be sure, biological control of pests, as distinguished from chemical control, is not a cut and dried affair. Many different approaches will have to be combined before the problems of pest control can be effectively resolved. But unless these methods are adopted and, above all, creatively integrated to suit the needs of each region, the use of pesticides will increase steadily in the years to come.

Another prevalent misconception about agriculture is that bigness *per se* makes for efficient and rational use of the land. The small farm has a potential advantage that the land factory and its close cousin, the plantation, seldom enjoy. A moderate-sized farm is dimensioned on a human scale. It lends itself to close scrutiny and careful management, to an intimacy between the farmer and the land that could engender a greater sensitivity to different soil needs and promote the employment of sound ecological practices. Small-scale farming could be successfully pursued as a form of applied ecology if blind economic interests were replaced with a sense of social responsibility. Unfortunately, many small farms in America are miniature replicas of the land factory. Agricultural units, large and small, tend to share the same ends—the "mass manufacture" of crops at the least cost.

A balanced system of food cultivation based on highly diversified, small-scale farms is not a utopian vision. The small farm still constitutes the backbone of agriculture in many areas of western Europe. Over many centuries heavy forest soils were slowly reconstructed to support livestock, orchards, and a large variety of field crops. Today, a diversified system of small-scale agriculture prevails in England, France, Scandinavia, and parts of West Germany. Most European farms, to be sure, are hardly models of good food cultivation; they often fail to make use of the ecological possibilities that exist in the moderate-sized agricultural unit. In contrast with most American farms, however, many European farms have created a workable relationship between man and the soil. These farms enjoy relatively high soil fertility despite centuries of use. Organic matter is often carefully returned to the land, and an entrenched tradition still resists the complete chemicalization of agriculture in many parts of England, France, and Germany.

So much for the dictates of ecology. If these dictates seem "unrealistic," it should be noted that in England today about 75 per cent of the farms have less than 300 acres and the average is about 100 acres. Agriculture in England and Wales has largely been stabilized around a small, highly diversified farming unit, almost equally divided between pasture and crop lands. Although many of these farms have been cultivated for 500 years or more, they have a far greater yield of wheat per acre than the average American agricultural unit and compare favorably with the latter in the output of other crops. American agriculture, driven by competition and an appetite for high earnings, is so much in flux that it is difficult to speak of sanity, still less of stability, in many rural areas of the United States. What is the trend? Robert S. McGlothin, of the Stanford Research Institute, suggests that by the end of the century, the number of American farms will have declined from 1.7 million to between 300,000 and 400,-000. These large argicultural units will produce about 90 per cent of the food cultivated in the United States. "Commercial farmsteads will be laid out and run like highly mechanized industrial plants. Crop and livestock production will be integrated into a comprehensive materials handling and marketing system. The independent family farmer will hire management counseling, which, with the aid of electronic computers, will help him program the operation of the entire farm system so as to achieve lowest unit costs of production. The computer will indicate—for each production season—which crops should be grown, where, in what quantities, when they should be fed to what livestock, and when and where marketed for greatest return."

To many, this may seem to be progress. To the ecologist, however, it represents an attempt to bring the laws of the biosphere into accordance with those of the market place, to reduce the natural world to merchandise. Nutritious crops can no more be expected to grow according to commercial schedules than man can be expected to adjust his pulse to the rhythm of machines.

CHAPTER EIGHT

Health and Society

INDIVIDUAL AND SOCIAL ASPECTS OF HEALTH

A NEW APPROACH is likely to gain easier acceptance if it involves individual rather than social action. The majority of people tend to look for immediate, practical solutions that they can adopt without having to face major social and environmental problems. They search for personal recipes and formulas for physical well-being. This attitude is understandable. Health and illness are intimate problems, involving the ability to survive and enjoy full lives. Health is enjoyed by the individual, not by such abstractions as "man" and "the community." Any discussion of health usually evokes the query: "What can I do right now to remove hazards to my health and assure my physical well-being?"

This question has been answered, to a great extent,

by authorities cited in the previous chapters—implicitly if not always directly. Diet should be highly varied. If at all possible, it should be based on foods that receive minimal or no treatment by processors, such as whole-wheat breads, fresh meat, vegetables, and fruit. Weight control is desirable in all stages of life, not only in middle age. Urban man should put his body to frequent use, with an emphasis on mild daily exercise, such as walking, rather than on sporadic sessions of competitive sports. Certainly smoking is utterly incompatible with good health and should be reduced or eliminated.

There is a good deal of evidence to indicate that a high intake of starches, sugars, and polysaturated fats predisposes the individual to coronary heart disease. At any rate, a diet that is ordinarily regarded as suitable for active growing children seems to be very undesirable for adults.* The food intake of the individual should be carefully scaled to his age, to his work load, and to his activities during leisure hours.

The individual should attempt to cultivate a serene attitude toward the surrounding world, an outlook based not on a psychoanalytic accommodation to the ills of society, but rather on a critical sense of values that places the trivia of daily life in a manageable perspective. To seek an uncritical, brainless state of euphoria is self-debasing. On the other hand, to respond with equal sensi-

---

* Let us pause to note that as little as fifteen or twenty years ago any plea for a reduction in the intake of eggs and dairy fats would have been furiously denounced by most nutritionists as "cultism" and "food faddism." Nutritionists tend to form ironclad opinions that are difficult to alter without long, often heated controversy; it is not uncommon to find nutritionists who still regard the dietary suggestions of Ancel and Margaret Keys in *Eat Well and Stay Well* as being a hairbreadth away from "quackery." The study of the human diet and its effects on health would benefit immensely if more investigators were willing to follow less conventional and more independent lines of inquiry.

tivity to every disquieting aspect of daily life is spiritually paralyzing and physically harmful. In trying to reduce the tensions that an overly urbanized, bitterly competitive society engenders in the individual, there is no substitute for a truly humanistic philosophy that helps us to discriminate between problems that warrant a strong emotional response and those that should be dismissed as inconsequential. To live a life without intense feeling is as dehumanizing as to live one that is filled with ill-defined, persistent agitation.

Health is the result of a lifelong process. It cannot be acquired by a pill or by a "magic" food. Physical well-being presupposes a rounded mode of life and a comprehensive diet geared to the needs of the body. Any attempt to prescribe a single "health-giving" recipe that fails to encompass the totality of the individual—his past as well as his present—is irresponsible. Neither "royal jelly" at one extreme nor a "miracle drug" at the other will provide an individual with health if his environment and manner of life are deteriorating. Attempts to resolve health into a single formula may be well-meaning, but they are woefully incomplete.

The need for a comprehensive approach to health is stressed in Iago Galdston's critique of modern medicine and his argument for social medicine. Modern medicine has failed, in Galdston's opinion, not because it has "no cure for cancer, for essential hypertension, or for multiple sclerosis. Were it to achieve these and other cures besides, it still would have failed." Its failure is due to the fact that "modern medicine is almost entirely preoccupied with diseases and with their treatment, and very little, if at all, with health. It is obvious that an individual sick with pneumococcus pneumonia can be effectively treated by chemo-therapeutic agents, or by antibiotics. But such an individual, though cured of his pneumonia, may, and most likely will, remain a sick man unless, in addition, efforts are made to help him regain his health." Galdston advocates more than convalescent care. He proposes a change in medical education, medical outlook, and medical methods. A physician trained according to the principles of social medicine "would not be moved to inquire 'what's he got and what's good for it,' but, confronted by an ailing individual, he would attempt to determine the nature and extent of the disability as it is manifest, not merely in the presenting symptoms, but in the over-all performance of the individual according to his position in life; that is, in the light of his age, educational, vocational, social, and other prerogatives and obligations. He would not affirm 'this man has a peptic ulcer,' and undertake to treat the ulcer, but would by the presence of the ulcer recognize that the individual is sick and seek to determine and to correct, or amend, what ails the individual; what, in other words, impedes the individual in the fulfillment of his adventure in living."

Galdston's remarks constitute a much-needed attempt to widen the contemporary medical outlook. Efforts to expand prevailing notions of illness, treatment, and health beyond the germ theory and the emphasis on specific cures for specific diseases were thwarted at the turn of the century. This defeat culminated in tragedy when Max von Pettenkofer, the great German sanitarian, took his life in 1901 in despair over the rejection of his viewpoint. Pettenkofer had never denied the germ theory of disease, regardless of popularizations of medical history to the contrary. The controversy in his time centered around whether germs alone caused disease or whether environmental conditions and the constitution of the individual should also be considered in the study of individual illness and epidemics. As John Shaw Billings, the great American authority on public health, put it in 1883: "It is important to remember . . . that the mere introduction of germs into the living organism does not ensure their multiplication, or the production of disease. The condition of the organism itself has much influence on the result. . . . Pasteur has certainly made a hasty generalization in declaring that the only condition which determines an epidemic is the greater or less abundance of germs."

Today, three generations later, the issue is being raised again—and in what appears to be a much broader sense than even Galdston has suggested. Many of the biological problems created by poor sanitation and slums have been resolved, at least in the Western world. We are no longer as deeply concerned with killing epidemics of communicable diseases as were Pasteur, Pettenkofer, and Billings. But we are very much concerned with harmful environmental influences on some of the most intimate aspects of individual life. The necessities of life, even its pleasures, are now being manufactured for the millions. As a nation of urban dwellers in a mass society, we are becoming increasingly dependent upon the decisions of others for the quality of our food, clothing, and shelter. These decisions affect not only our diet and our private lives; they affect the water we drink and the air we breathe. To speak of an environmental "influence" on health is an understatement; there is a distinct environmental and social dimension to every aspect of human biology. Man today is more domesticated than he has ever been in the long course of his history.

It is here that we encounter the limits of the individual's ability to attain health on his own. The average man finds it extremely difficult to reorganize his mode of life along lines that favor well-being and fitness. If he lives in the city, he cannot possibly avoid exposure to air pollutants. Similarly, there are hardly any rural areas in America where the individual is not exposed to the assortment of pesticides that are currently employed in agriculture. Any serious attempt to limit the diet to pure foods, free of pesticide residues, artificial coloring and flavoring matter, and synthetic preservatives, is well beyond the financial means of the average person. But even if the individual can afford it, he will find that untreated foods are difficult to obtain, for relatively few pure foods are grown in the United States and those that reach urban centers are rarely sold in large retail markets. The layout of the modern city and its routine demands on the urban dweller tend to discourage a physically active way of life. Movement in the large city is organized around the automobile and public means of transportation. Most of our occupations and responsibilities demand mental dexterity, a routine of limited physical work, or rapid communication. It requires a heroic effort to walk instead of ride, to do instead of see, to move instead of sit. Although a few exceptional individuals may succeed in modifying their mode of life in a way that promotes health, the overwhelming majority of urban dwellers can be expected to go along with things as they are.

Does this mean that modern man will never attain optimal health, that it is, in fact, a "mirage"? Rene Dubos has argued rather persuasively that health is a relative concept. Man's criteria of health change with the economic, cultural, and political goals of each social period. "Clearly, health and disease cannot be defined merely in terms of anatomical, physiological, or mental attributes," Dubos writes. "Their real measure is the ability of the individual to function in a manner acceptable to himself and to the group of which he is part. . . . For several centuries the Western world has pretended to find a unifying concept of health in the Greek ideal of a proper balance between body and mind. But in reality this ideal is more and more difficult to convert into practice. Poets, philosophers, and creative scientists are rarely found among Olympic laureates. It is not easy to discover a formula of health broad enough to fit Voltaire and Jack Dempsey, to encompass the requirements of a stevedore, a New York City bus driver, and a contemplative monk."

Perhaps so. But the truth is not exhausted by the limited notions men form of a given event or situation. That which individuals, classes, or communities really believe to be health in a given historical period—all pretensions aside—does not tell us what health *could* be or what it *should* be in a broader biological and social perspective. It is one thing to say that historical notions of health have been limited; it is quite another to contend that they will always be limited. Although Dubos may be correct in describing life as a series of ideals for which men can be expected to sacrifice their health and even their lives, there is no reason to believe that health, defined primarily "in terms of anatomical, physiological, or mental attributes," is incompatible with a rational manner of life. On the contrary, a manner of life that promotes health is likely to be more satisfying culturally and socially than one that militates against the attainment of fitness and well-being. Health is nourished by all the environmental and social factors that advance thought, creative effort, and a rounded personality. The social factors that promote health also promote the adventure of life.

On the other hand, the more cloistered the man, the more cloistered the mind. The more one-sided the way of life, however "challenging" or "adventurous" it may seem on the surface, the more limited the range of thought and art. Voltaire was a brilliant writer but a superficial thinker. His life, spent for the most part at the château of Cirey and in his "lairs" on the Franco-Swiss border, shows in his work. One is entitled to wonder whether he would have acquired greater depth had he been exposed, like his more profound contemporary, Diderot, to an earthier life in the streets of Paris. Similarly, Olympic laureates seldom become poets and philosophers because their limited notions of "adventure" are focused entirely on physical activity for its own sake. Far from challenging the "Greek ideal of a proper balance between body and mind," the very incompleteness of their lives and thought is evidence of its validity.

Dubos, in effect, tends to equate health with adaptation. The environments to which men are expected to adapt are conceived of as dynamic, emergent phenomena —a rather ambiguous approach that seems to take the environment too much for granted. Unlike other animals, man can consciously remake his environment, within certain limits, and the real issue to be faced is whether it is man or his unsatisfactory environment that should be changed. Viewed from this standpoint, the problem becomes much clearer. One can conceive of many circumstances in which health is not an end in itself and even of circumstances in which the achievement of certain ends is worth the loss of health. By and large, however, a health-promoting environment encourages social and cultural progress. There need be no conflict between health and a truly creative, rational civilization.

On the whole, however, Dubos has performed a notable service in focusing attention on the relationship between human fitness and social development. We cannot conceive of progress in the field of public health without advances in society. Management of the soil has always depended upon the prevailing forms of land tenure. The quality of today's food is partly determined by whether the interests of food manufacturers or the interests of consumers determine technological changes in the industry. The form and direction taken by urban life are guided by the kind of social relations men establish in the management of their affairs. Any attempt to preserve the health of individuals which does not also aim at creating social patterns that will favor the health of mankind as a whole may result in limited improvement but not long-range solutions. The majority of individuals who seek optimal health as soloists in a deteriorating environment have far too much to cope with in attaining their ends.

At the same time, today, more than at any other time in history, every social change has deep-seated biological consequences. Man has developed extremely effective methods for changing the world around him. The results of his activity over the face of the earth are far-reaching. The natural world can no longer successfully oppose dense forests, vast bodies of water, and climatic rigors to his penetration. The developments of modern technology have deprived nature of its old defenses against the invasion of man. But the natural world can strike back in the form of disease, exhaustion of the soil, and desiccation of the land. The importance of caution and the need for exercising reason in changing the world around us can hardly be given too much emphasis. "What is new is not necessarily good," Dubos observes, "and all changes, even those apparently the most desirable, are always fraught with unpredictable consequences. The scientist must beware of having to admit, like Captain Ahab in Melville's *Moby Dick,* 'All my means are sane; my motives and objects mad.' "

THE PROBLEMS OF REMEDIAL LEGISLATION

How MUCH PROGRESS can we expect from attempts to improve the health of the American public by means of legislation? More, certainly, than we can expect from isolated individual efforts. The United States has by no means exhausted all the possibilities of welfare legislation; it has lagged behind many European nations in fulfilling its responsibilities to the sick and the infirm. Its national health programs consist of *ad hoc* aid and a patchwork of laboratories and clinics to meet the mounting needs of research and therapy. Food and drug laws have not kept pace with the rapid changes in food technology, and the operations of federal agencies responsible for administering them leave much to be desired. An account of the advances, conflicts, and retreats in the field of food and drug control offers a valuable perspective on what remedial legislation can and cannot be expected to do.

The problems of food and drug control have been surrounded by such a dense fog of official overstatement that almost any criticism of existing laws and agencies invites countercharges of "quackery" and "faddism." Consider the following blurb, made up in part of official statements, which the public is expected to accept as good coin:

"When the American housewife pushes her shopping cart through the supermarket, she can select attractively packaged foods and drinks with the confidence that they are honestly labeled, pure and wholesome. Her confidence is based on the existence of good laws that are vigilantly enforced. Most American food manufacturers today have the will and the know-how to produce the pure foods that she wants. They accept the Food, Drug, and Cosmetic Act as a blueprint of their obligations to the Nation's consumers. The additives that go into food are there to improve the food and bring it to the housewife in better condition and in a more convenient form. Reliable food processors have not reduced the nutritional quality of our foods or created inferior products through the use of chemical additives. Actually, the quality and sanitary characteristics of our food have been improving."

Most of these complacent remarks can be dismissed as rubbish. Without doing any injustice to the facts, the blurb might be rewritten as follows:

"When the American housewife pushes her shopping cart through the supermarket, she encounters many products whose packaging often misleads her concerning the quality, quantity, and nutritive value of their contents. Generally, the enforcement of food-labeling laws and regulations has been handled in a very slovenly fashion by federal and state authorities. Most processed foods are certainly not 'pure,' if by a pure product is meant one that does not contain chemical additives. Food and drug control is far from satisfactory, and it has often been necessary to prod federal agencies into discharging their responsibilities to the consumer. The F.D.A. has shown an unusual susceptibility to influence from the food industry; the agency's performance has been distinguished by its leniency and patience with food manufacturers. More often than not, food processors and drug manufacturers have bitterly opposed improvements in regulatory legislation. Although some of the chemicals that are added to food may possibly improve them, the safety of many food additives is very doubtful. Finally, reliable food manufacturers have definitely reduced the nutritive value of certain common foods, and additives have often served to conceal inferior products."

The first statement attempts to evade the problems of modern food control; the second, to face them. It is almost begging the question to claim that producers of food accept the Food, Drug, and Cosmetic Act as "a blueprint of their obligations to the Nation's consumers" when the law is not as demanding as it should be and those who administer it are satisfied with a second-rate achievement.

Nor is the case for the law strengthened by smuggling the housewife's "wants" into the issue. The wants of many consumers are created by high-pressure advertising and salesmanship. The average consumer knows far too little about nutrition to evaluate advertising claims. Food purchases are guided partly by sales technique, partly by the appearance of the food. Thus, the food industry tends to generate the very wants it professes to satisfy, and conventional books and articles on nutrition tend to equate the satisfaction of these industry-created wants with improvements in the quality and purity of our food.

The truth is that federal food and drug legislation has always been a poor, unstable compromise between the interests of the food industry and the demands of an aroused public opinion. More than a quarter of a century separates the first unsuccessful attempts to enact a general anti-adulteration law (1879) and the adoption of the basic Food and Drug Law of 1906. The story behind these and later conflicts in the field of pure-food legislation indicates the amount of effort that has been required to preserve the integrity of our food supply. The needs of industry were consistently given priority over those of the public; during this entire period, Congress was quick to favor special interests. It put an end to the export of adulterated products only when the reputation of American food began to decline on the world market. It enacted legislation against oleomargarine in behalf of domestic dairy interests. On the whole, the public interest was served only indirectly. At the turn of the century, the most flagrant cases of adulteration were the work of small-scale producers, whose adulterated goods placed major producers at a competitive disadvantage. In these cases, both Congress and most of the food manufacturers responded readily to the need for specific anti-adulteration legislation, but the food industry's support for a general food law was, at best, hesitant, and in the halls of Congress support for a pure-food law gathered very slowly.

It is extremely doubtful whether any general food and drug legislation would have been adopted in 1906 were it not for the efforts of Harvey W. Wiley and the unexpected support his efforts received from the publication of Upton Sinclair's *The Jungle*, a novel which criticized the social and sanitary conditions in the Chicago stockyards. Wiley was a gifted physician and chemist whose pioneering research in sugar, soil, and food analysis brought him to the position of chief of the U. S. Department of Agriculture's Bureau of Chemistry. His prestige as a scientist, his Hoosier wit, and his engaging personality gained him wide professional and public admiration. The task of ensuring a pure food supply for the American consumer became Wiley's life work. His lectures, articles, reports, and congressional testimony mobilized widely disparate groups—from urban civic clubs to farm organizations—behind the demand for a general anti-adulteration law. The food industry at first followed Wiley cautiously, later reluctantly, and finally, with few exceptions, turned against him. In the spring of 1906, when the issue reached its climax in Congress, opposition from the food industry nearly succeeded in preventing the enactment of an effective pure food and drug law. As late as June 1906, after much wrangling in the House of Representatives, Wiley despaired of getting a law. "No serious attempts, so far as I know," he wrote, "have been made to set a date for its consideration."

The publication of *The Jungle* in book form (January 1906), however, had aroused widespread public indignation against the meat-packing industry. The scales were tipped in favor of the law when President Theodore Roosevelt released part of a report by a federal investigating commission which fully corroborated the details in Sinclair's novel. The national uproar that followed these disclosures threw the industry into retreat, and on June 30, 1906, the first federal Pure Food and Drug Act was signed into law. Its administration was placed largely in the hands of Wiley and his Bureau of Chemistry. Although the law had many shortcomings, some of which were corrected in later years, the high standards of food and drug control which Wiley sought to establish during his tenure in office have never been equaled by his successors. The history of the fight for pure food after Wiley's departure from government service reads like an anticlimax to the vigilance and dedication that marked earlier policies.

These policies were guided by two basic principles. The first was that the consumer should know precisely what he is getting and that he should get precisely what he wants. Wiley bitterly opposed labels or claims that misrepresented a product to the buyer, even if the use of a spurious description was harmless to public health. He stubbornly fought attempts by food manufacturers to describe glucose as "corn syrup" or to represent whiskey made partly of neutral grain spirits as "blended whiskey," a name that generally denoted a blend of several genuine whiskeys. For Wiley, a label had to be complete and truthful. He expected the food manufacturer to disclose all the artificial ingredients added to a product. The name on a package, can, or bottle had to convey the nature of the product without any ambiguity or misrepresentation.

Wiley's second principle was that if any doubt exists about the toxicity of a chemical additive, the doubt should be resolved in favor of the consumer. As it is impossible to prove a negative such as "harmlessness," Wiley argued, it is not permissible to use any questionable additive that is not indispensable to the production, storage, or distribution of food. If an additive contributed nothing to health

or to the availability of a food, and if its use might conceivably prove harmful, the Bureau of Chemistry sought
to have it removed. Wiley seldom wavered on this score;
his decisions almost invariably favored the public interest.

Many people in the food and chemical industries felt
differently, however, and their complaints evoked a sympathetic response from the government. By 1912, Wiley's
attempts to execute his policies were being frustrated to
such an extent that he left government service. With his
departure, the law underwent steady reinterpretation. An
increasing number of doubts about the toxicity of new
chemical additives were resolved in favor of food growers
and food processors. The Bureau of Chemistry and its suc-
cessor in the enforcement of the law, the Food and Drug
Administration, began to exhibit undue sensitivity to the
financial welfare of industry. The improvement of food
was equated with lower costs, attractive packaging, and
sales-promotion devices. Wiley had combined the zeal of
a crusader with the knowledge of a physician; with his
departure, the policies of the federal regulatory agencies
were guided increasingly by lawyers and professional ad-
ministrators who began to give priority to legal considerations instead of problems of public health.

The consumer could ill afford this development. Although an overhaul of the food and drug law was made in
1938, the situation began to deteriorate to an appalling
extent. After the end of World War II, the American food
supply was deluged with an unprecedented variety of
new chemical additives. DDT and other organic insecticides, unknown in 1938, were being used extensively in
agriculture and the home. The responsibility for proving
that a chemical additive was harmful to the consumer
rested with the F.D.A. Food growers and food processors
were free to use what they chose until such time as the
government could establish that the additives involved

were toxic substances. Testing standards in many laboratories were inadequate; experimental work on new additives was often limited to sixty- and ninety-day feeding trials on one or two species of rodents.

In September 1958, Congress changed the law drastically; it made the manufacturer responsible for establishing the safety of a food additive and inserted the Delaney anti-cancer clause, a provision that flatly prohibits the use of additives "found to induce cancer when ingested by man or animal . . ." Although the anti-cancer clause was strongly supported by the American Cancer Society and by leading cancer specialists, it was opposed by the F.D.A. Testifying in April 1958 before a House committee studying pending revisions of the law, F.D.A. Commissioner George P. Larrick observed: "Two of the bills before you make specific mention of cancer." The F.D.A.-supported bill, H.R. 6747, does "not mention it specifically . . . This bill bars the use of an additive unless it is established that it is without hazard to health. Thus, the bill would prohibit the addition of any chemical additive to the food supply until adequate evidence, acceptable to competent scientists, shows that it will not produce cancer in man under the conditions of use proposed." Although Larrick endorsed the goal of "seeing that cancer-producing foods are not on the American market," Congressman Delaney reminded the National Health Federation that "in 1956 an FDA ruling permitted, at a certain concentration, residues of a pesticide to remain on marketed fruits and vegetables, even though it had been shown to induce cancer in test animals. Later tests showed this chemical to be even more injurious than the earlier tests demonstrated, and the FDA has now taken action to prohibit any of its residues on raw agricultural commodities."

The credit for finally adding an anti-cancer clause to

the 1958 law must be given to Delaney, who saw to its enactment despite strong opposition from the food industry and the F.D.A. By 1960, the F.D.A. had reversed its position and, at the hearings on food colors conducted by the House Committee on Interstate and Foreign Commerce, expressed its fervent support for the Delaney clause. Presumably all is well that ends well, but the F.D.A. refuses to let the clause remain as it is. At the food-color hearings, the Secretary of Health, Education, and Welfare, Arthur S. Flemming, began to nibble at the Delaney clause by suggesting that it "should be modified to provide that additives used in animal feed which leave no residue either in the animal after slaughter or in any food product obtained from the living animal be exempt from the provisions of the clause. A comparable amendment to the anti-cancer clause in the color additive legislation under consideration would be appropriate." Experience with Yellow OB and Yellow AB suggests that such standards of purity are impossible to achieve (see page 139).

The sweeping legislative revisions of 1958 were not gained without a sacrifice. For all its shortcomings, the 1938 law had one redeeming feature: It flatly prohibited the use of any toxic chemical additives in food other than those that were clearly indispensable to food production. Although the burden of proof rested with the F.D.A. instead of the manufacturers, the 1938 law set a new functional standard for chemical additives in food. This criterion was dropped in the 1958 revisions of the law, largely on the urging of the food industry and the F.D.A. The burden of proving that the additives are safe has been shifted to the manufacturers, but toxic chemicals can now be added to food provided they are used in amounts that are deemed to be "harmless" to consumers.

Thus, after the passage of a half century, the law

makes no attempt to resolve Wiley's original problem: Does an additive contribute to the nutritive value and availability of a food or does it merely function as a dispensable technological aid? Modern refrigeration and canning techniques have eliminated the need for many artificial preservatives in our food supply. Hardly anyone will contend that coloring and flavoring matter are indispensable to food production. If consumers really desired artificial colors and flavors, they could be marketed as independent products and the public could use them at its own discretion. The food industry could modify its production methods so as to operate with a minimum number of chemical additives and with a view toward retaining many nutrients that are now lost because of an overemphasis on mass production and highly processed foods. Many synthetic additives that have no nutritive function could easily be replaced with valuable nutrients. For example, ascorbic acid (vitamin C) is a good antioxidant and an excellent flour bleach, but as it is relatively costly, it would be unprofitable to use it.

The food industry has demanded complete freedom in determining the function of chemical additives in food. The following remarks by the National Association of Frozen Food Packers are fairly typical: "We join with other segments of the food industry in fundamental opposition to provisions which would permit the Food and Drug Administration to determine the composition of food products upon the basis of its conception of functional value or utility of food ingredients." This seems to be a matter of principle, not a lack of confidence in the F.D.A. After asserting that the chances are "rather remote" that a food processor would engage in costly tests of a toxic additive, the association adds: "In any case, the question of usefulness of an ingredient shown to be safe is one which the manufacturer of a food is entitled to resolve upon the basis of his own experience, and is not properly a matter of the opinion of the Food and Drug Administration."

The F.D.A.'s superficial approach to food and drug legislation has largely been exhausted. The next overhaul of the law must return to the principles that guided Wiley a half century ago. Moreover, we require not only a better food and drug law but comprehensive national legislation that will confront the problems raised by urban and industrial pollution, radioactive contaminants, the misuse of X radiation, and industrial carcinogens. Water pollution can be appreciably reduced if all sizable communities are required to treat their sewage and if an effective national program is developed to reclaim and re-use water to meet industrial needs. The highest-quality water, that which requires a minimum of chemical treatment, should be reserved for drinking purposes. The problem of air pollution should be met resolutely, without qualms about cost and without fear of offending industrialists, motorists, or homeowners. Recently developed catalytic and non-catalytic burners, for example, can remove many harmful agents from automobile exhausts. "Automobile engineers know now that for perhaps $10 per car they can eliminate 50 per cent of the hydrocarbons; for something over $300 they can eliminate them almost totally," observes George A. W. Boehm, of *Fortune* magazine. "Any city or state that decides to apply air-pollution regulations to cars will have to decide how much the motorist can be made to pay for how much purity, and how far it is prepared to go in enforcing purity regulations."

But let us not deceive ourselves; an environment based on mammoth, expanding cities will never be a healthy one. In the United States, the ecological and nutritional problems created by monoculture and the land factory are likely to grow worse, and many chemical additives will be required in the mass production of our food. Insecticidal residues will undoubtedly continue to pervade our food staples. The substitution of nuclear energy for mineral sources of fuel will be accelerated in the years to come, and more radioactive substances can be expected to enter man's environment. Urban life will undoubtedly become increasingly one-sided as cities expand and occupations become more sedentary. The improvements that our technicians, sanitarians, and city planners have projected for the "world of tomorrow" may meliorate some of these problems, but they are not likely to eliminate them if our society continues to develop in the pattern of the giant metropolis. We can no more expect engineering devices to give us a healthful environment than we can expect the therapeutic agents of modern medicine to create a healthy individual.

DECENTRALIZATION

WITHOUT HAVING READ any books or articles on human ecology, millions of Americans have sensed the over-all deterioration of modern urban life. They have turned to the suburbs and "exurbs" as a refuge from the burdens of the metropolitan milieu. From all accounts of suburban life, many of these burdens have followed them into the countryside. Suburbanites have not adapted to the land; they have merely adapted a metropolitan manner of life to semi-rural surroundings. The metropolis remains the axis around which their lives turn. It is the source of their livelihood, their food staples, and, in large part, their tensions. The suburbs have branched away from the city, but they still belong to the metropolitan tree.

It would be wise, however, to stop ridiculing the

exodus to the suburbs and to try to understand what lies behind this phenomenon. The modern city has reached its limits. Megalopolitan life is breaking down—psychically, economically, and biologically. Millions of people have acknowledged this breakdown by "voting with their feet"; they have picked up their belongings and left. If they have not been able to sever their connections with the metropolis, at least they have tried. As a social symptom, the effort is significant. The reconciliation of man with the natural world is no longer merely desirable; it has become a necessity. It is a compelling need that is sending millions of people into the countryside. The need has created a new interest in camping, handicrafts, and horticulture. In ever-increasing numbers, Americans are acquiring a passionate interest in their national parks and forests, in their rural landscape, and in their small-town agrarian heritage.

Despite its many shortcomings, this trend reflects a basically sound orientation. The average American is making an attempt, however confusedly, to reduce his environment to a human scale. He is trying to re-create a world that he can cope with as an individual, a world that he correctly identifies with the freedom, gentler rhythms, and quietude of rural surroundings. His attempts at gardening, landscaping, carpentry, home maintenance, and other so-called suburban "vices" reflect a need to function within an intelligible, manipulatable, and individually creative sphere of human activity. The suburbanite, like the camper, senses that he is working with basic, abiding things that have slipped from his control in the metropolitan world—shelter, the handiwork that enters into daily life, vegetation, and the land. He is fortunate, to be sure, if these activities do not descend to the level of caricature. Nevertheless, they are important, not only because they reflect basic needs of man but because they also reflect basic needs of the things with which he is working. The human scale is also the natural scale. The soil, the land, the living things on which man depends for his nutriment and recreation are direly in need of individual care.

For one thing, proper maintenance of the soil not only depends upon advances in our knowledge of soil chemistry and soil fertility; it also requires a more personalized approach to agriculture. Thus far, the trend has been the other way; agriculture has become depersonalized and over-industrialized. Modern farming is suffering from gigantism. The average agricultural unit is getting so big that the finer aspects of soil performance and soil needs are being overlooked. If differences in the quality and performance of various kinds of soil are to receive more attention, American farming must be reduced to a more human scale. It will become necessary to bring agriculture within the scope of the individual, so that the farmer and the soil can develop together, each responding as fully as possible to the needs of the other.

The same is true for the management of livestock. Today our food animals are being manipulated like a lifeless industrial resource. Normally, large numbers of animals are collected in the smallest possible area and are allowed only as much movement as is necessary for mere survival. Our meat animals have been placed on a diet composed for the most part of medicated feed high in carbohydrates. Before they are slaughtered, these obese, rapidly matured creatures seldom spend more than six months on the range and six months on farms, where they are kept on concentrated rations and gain about two pounds daily. Our dairy herds are handled like machines; our poultry flocks, like hothouse tomatoes. The need to restore the time-honored intimacy between man and his livestock is just as pronounced as the need to bring agriculture within the horizon of the individual farmer. Although modern technology has enlarged the elements that enter into the agricultural situation, giving each man a wider area of sovereignty and control, machines have not lessened the importance of personal familiarity with the land, its vegetation, and the living things it supports. Unless principles of good land use permit otherwise, a farm should not become smaller or larger than the individual farmer can command. If it is smaller, agriculture will become inefficient; if larger, it will become depersonalized.

With the decline in the quality of urban life, on the one hand, and the growing imbalance in agriculture, on the other, our times are beginning to witness a remarkable confluence of human interests with the needs of the natural world. Men of the nineteenth century assumed a posture of defiance toward the forests, plains, and mountains. Their applause was reserved for the engineer, the technician, the inventor, at times even the robber baron and the railroader, who seemed to offer the promise of a more abundant material life. Today we are filled with a vague nostalgia for the past. To a large degree this nostalgia reflects the insecurity and uncertainty of our times, in contrast with the echoes of a more optimistic and perhaps more tranquil era. But it also reflects a deep sense of loss, a longing for the free, unblemished land that lay before the eyes of the frontiersman and early settler. We are seeking out the mountains they tried to avoid and we are trying to recover fragments of the forests they removed. Our nostalgia springs neither from a greater sensitivity nor from the wilder depths of human instinct. It springs from a growing need to restore the normal, balanced, and manageable rhythms of human life—that is, an environment that meets our requirements as individuals and biological beings.

Modern man can never return to the primitive life he so often idealizes, but the point is that he doesn't have to. The use of farm machinery as such does not conflict with sound agricultural practices; nor are industry and an urbanized community incompatible with a more agrarian, more natural environment. Ironically, advances in technology itself have largely overcome the industrial problems that once justified the huge concentrations of people and facilities in a few urban areas. Automobiles, aircraft, electric power, and electronic devices have eliminated nearly all the problems of transportation, communication, and social isolation that burdened man in past eras. We can now communicate with one another over a distance of thousands of miles in a matter of seconds, and we can travel to the most remote areas of the world in a few hours. The obstacles created by space and time are essentially gone. Similarly, size need no longer be a problem. Technologists have developed remarkable small-scale alternatives to many of the giant facilities that still dominate modern industry. The smoky steel town, for example, is an anachronism. Excellent steel can be made and rolled with installations that occupy about two or three city blocks.* Many of the latest machines are highly versatile and compact. They lend themselves to a large variety of manufacturing and finishing operations. Today the more modern plant, with its clean, quiet, versatile, and largely automated facilities, contrasts sharply with the huge, ugly, congested factories inherited from an earlier industrial era.

Thus, almost without realizing it, we have been pre-

---

* For example, by using Sendzimir's planetary rolling mill, which reduces a 2¼-inch-thick steel slab to ⅒ of an inch in a single pass through a set of work rolls. The conventional continuous strip mill involves the use of scale-breaker stands, about four roughening stands, six finishing stands, long roller tables, and other machines —a huge and costly installation.

paring the material conditions for a new type of human community—one which constitutes neither a complete return to the past nor a suburban accommodation to the present. It is no longer fanciful to think of man's future environment in terms of a decentralized, moderate-sized city that combines industry with agriculture, not only in the same civic entity but in the occupational activities of the same individual. The "urbanized farmer" or the "agrarianized townsman" need not be a contradiction in terms. This way of life was achieved for a time by the Greek polis, by early republican Rome, and by the Renaissance commune. The urban centers that became the well-springs of Western civilization were not strictly cities, in the modern sense of the term. Rather, they brought agriculture together with urban life, synthesizing both into a rounded human, cultural, and social development.

Whether modern man manages to reach this point or travels only part of the way, some kind of decentralization will be necessary to achieve a lasting equilibrium between society and nature. Urban decentralization underlies any hope of achieving ecological control of pest infestations in agriculture. Only a community well integrated with the resources of the surrounding region can promote agricultural and biological diversity. With careful planning, man could use plants and animals not only as a source of food but also, by pitting one species of life against another, as a means of controlling pests, thus eliminating much of his need for chemical methods. What is equally important, a decentralized community holds the greatest promise for conserving natural resources, particularly as it would promote the use of local sources of energy. Instead of relying primarily on concentrated sources of fuel in distant regions of the continent, the community could make maximum use of its own energy resources, such as wind power, solar energy, and hydroelectric power. These sources of energy, so often overlooked because of an almost exclusive reliance on a national division of labor, would help greatly to conserve the remaining supply of high-grade petroleum and coal. They would almost certainly postpone, if not eliminate, the need for turning to radioactive substances and nuclear reactors as major sources of industrial energy. With more time at his disposal for intensive research, man might learn either to employ solar energy and wind power as the principal sources of energy or to eliminate the hazard of radioactive contamination from nuclear reactors.

It is true, of course, that our life lines would become more complex and, from a technological point of view, less "efficient." There would be many duplications of effort. Instead of being concentrated in two or three areas of the country, steel plants would be spread out, with many communities employing small-scale facilities to meet regional or local needs. But the word "efficiency," like the word "pest," is a relative term. Although a duplication of facilities would be somewhat costly, many local mineral sources that are not used today because they are too widely scattered or too small for the purposes of large-scale production, would become economical for the purposes of a smaller community. Thus, in the long run, a more localized or regional form of industrial activity is likely to promote a more efficient use of resources than our prevailing methods of production.

It is true that we will never entirely eliminate the need for a national and international division of labor in agriculture and industry. The Midwest will always remain the best source of our grains; the East and Far West, the best sources of lumber and certain field crops. Our petroleum, high-grade coal, and certain minerals will still have to be supplied, in large part, by a few regions of the country. But there is no reason why we cannot reduce the burden that our national division of labor currently places on these areas by spreading the agricultural and industrial loads over wider areas of the country. This seems to be the only approach to the task of creating a long-range balance between man and the natural world and of remaking man's synthetic environment in a form that will promote human health and fitness.

An emphasis on agriculture and urban regionalism is somewhat disconcerting to the average city dweller. It conjures up an image of cultural isolation and social stagnation, of a journey backward in history to the agrarian societies of the medieval and ancient worlds. Actually, the urban dweller today is more isolated in the big city than his ancestors were in the countryside. The city man in the modern metropolis has reached a degree of anonymity, social atomization, and spiritual isolation that is virtually unprecedented in human history. Today man's alienation from man is almost absolute. His standards of co-operation, mutual aid, simple human hospitality, and decency have suffered an appalling amount of erosion in the urban milieu. Man's civic institutions have become cold, impersonal agencies for the manipulation of his destiny, and his culture has increasingly accommodated itself to the least common denominator of intelligence and taste. He has nothing to lose even by a backward glance; indeed, in this way he is likely to place his present-day world and its limitations in a clearer perspective.

But why should an emphasis on agriculture and urban regionalism be regarded as an attempt to return to the past? Can we not develop our environment more selectively, more subtly, and more rationally than we have thus far, combining the best of the past and present and bringing forth a new synthesis of man and nature, nation and region, town and country? Life would indeed cease to be an adventure if we merely elaborated the present by extending urban sprawl and by expanding civic life until it completely escapes from the control of its individual human elements. To continue along these lines would serve not to promote social evolution but rather to "fatten" the social organism to a point where it could no longer move. Our purpose should be to make individual life a more rounded experience, and this we can hope to accomplish at the present stage of our development only by restoring the complexity of man's environment and by reducing the community to a human scale.

Is there any evidence that reason will prevail in the management of our affairs? It is difficult to give a direct answer. Certainly we are beginning to look for qualitative improvements in many aspects of life; we are getting weary and resentful of the shoddiness in our goods and services. We are gaining a new appreciation of the land and its problems, and a greater realization of the social promise offered by a more manageable human community. More and more is being written about our synthetic environment, and the criticism is more pointed than it has been in almost half a century. Perhaps we can still hope, as Mumford did more than two decades ago in the closing lines of *The Culture of Cities:*

"We have much to unbuild, and much more to build: but the foundations are ready: the machines are set in place and the tools are bright and keen: the architects, the engineers, and the workmen are assembled. None of us may live to see the complete building, and perhaps in the nature of things the building can never be completed: but some of us will see the flag or the fir tree that the workers will plant aloft in ancient ritual when they cap the topmost story."

I T WOULD require an enormous amount of space to cite the many works that directly helped to form the views presented in this book. Some measure of discrimination and selection has been necessary. Wherever possible, the author has cited a source that offers generalizations or a reasonably comprehensive review of experimental data. In many cases, however, it has been necessary to adduce the original papers in which the results of a research project appeared. Although the professional literature in medical journals seldom falls within the purview of the general reader, it has seemed wisest to document many points that are currently in dispute, particularly in regard to such emotionally charged issues as food additives, environmental cancer, and ionizing radiation.

The references preceding the following notes indicate the line at which the passage in question begins—the beginning of a quotation, the opening words of a sentence containing a particular statement of fact, or the point at which an extensive discussion begins.

Chapter One: The Problem

p. 4, l. 20   Philip M. Hauser: *Population Perspectives* (New Brunswick, N.J.: Rutgers University Press; 1961), p. 98, Table 17; also pp. 96-8.

p. 4, l. 30   Herman E. Kroose: *American Economic Development* (Englewood Cliffs, N.J.: Prentice-Hall, Inc.; 1957), p. 179.

p. 5, l. 19   "Change in Rank of Leading Causes of Death," *Statistical Bulletin*, Metropolitan Life Insurance Co., Vol. 31, No. 6 (1950), p. 8. U. S. Public Health Service: *Death Rates by Age, Race, and Sex, United States, 1900-1953, Vital Statistics—Special Reports*, Vol. 43, Nos. 2, 11, 12, 13, 14, 15, 16, 17, 18, and 19 (Washington: U. S. Government Printing Office; 1956).

p. 5, l. 32   Cf. U. S. Public Health Service: *Health Statistics from the U. S. National Health Survey, July 1957-June 1958*, Series B: Nos. 12, 13, 20, and Series C: Nos. 5, 6 (Washington: U. S. Government Printing Office; 1959, 1960).

p. 6, l. 21   W. C. Hueper: "Age Aspects of Environmental and Occupational Cancers," *Public Health Reports*, Vol. 67 (1952), p. 774. Harold F. Dorn and Sidney J. Cutler: *Morbidity from Cancer in the United States*, U. S. Public Health Service, Public Health Monograph No. 56 (Washington: U. S. Government Printing Office; 1959), pp. 52-3.

p. 7, l. 3   Unpublished data furnished to the author by the American Cancer Society; compiled from *Vital Statistics of the United States*.

p. 7, l. 35   William F. Enos *et al.*: "Coronary Disease among United States Soldiers Killed in Action in Korea," *Journal of the American Medical Association*, Vol. 152 (1953), p. 1090.

p. 8, l. 18   Ira Gore *et al.*: "Coronary Atherosclerosis and Myocardial Infarction in Kyusha, Japan, and Boston, Massachusetts," *Proceedings of the New England Cardiovascular Society*, 1961-2, Vol. 19 (in press).

p. 8, l. 22   According to a recent report in the *Medical Tribune*, for example, Jerome Samuel and Bernard Weiss, of the Polyclinic Medical School and Hospital in New York City, find a "'sharply increased trend in [gastric] ulcers' in the four-to-twelve age group, even allowing for the facts of greater awareness of the possibility and improved diagnostic techniques." "Peptic Ulcers Found Increasing in Young from 4-12 Years Old," *Medical Tribune*, Vol. 2, No. 29 (1961), p. 16.

p. 9, l. 16   Lester A. Breslow: "Exposure to Low Concentrations of Air Pollution (1)—Health Effects from Repeated Exposure," *Proceedings of the National Conference on Air Pollution* (Washington: U. S. Government Printing Office; 1959), p. 197.

p. 9, footnote   Sloan-Kettering Institute for Cancer Research: *Progress Report XI*, New York (1958), pp. 11-13.

p. 10, footnote   Iago Galdston: *The Meaning of Social Medicine* (Cambridge, Mass.: Harvard University Press; 1954), p. 57.

p. 11, l. 15   Cf. Rene and Jean Dubos: *The White Plague* (Boston: Little, Brown & Company; 1952).

p. 14, l. 1   Cf. Norman Jolliffe: "Obesity—Its Prevalence, Etiology, Effects on Health, Management," *Proceedings of the National Food and Nutrition Institute*, December 8, 9, 10, 1952, U. S. Department of Agriculture, Agricultural Handbook No. 56, pp. 73-4. "Frequency of Overweight and Underweight," *Statistical Bulletin,* Metropolitan Life Insurance Co., Vol. 41, No. 1 (1960), pp. 4-7.

p. 14, l. 7 L. Jean Bogert: *Nutrition and Physical Fitness* (Philadelphia: W. B. Saunders Company; 1960), pp. 319-20.

p. 14, l. 14 According to Katz, Stammler, and Pick, there has been a substantial increase in the intake of fatty foods in the United States. Cf. L. N. Katz *et al.*: "Nutritional and Atherosclerosis," *Federation Proceedings,* Vol. 15 (1956), p. 889.

p. 14, l. 30 Norman Jolliffe: *Reduce and Stay Reduced* (New York: Simon & Schuster; 1957), pp. 22-3. There is now an impressive body of evidence to support this conclusion. Cf. Albert Tannenbaum: "Relationship of Body Weight to Cancer Incidence," *A.M.A. Archives of Pathology,* Vol. 30 (1940), pp. 509-17. Albert Tannenbaum: "Effects of Varying Caloric Intake upon Tumor Incidence and Tumor Growth," *Annals of the New York Academy of Science,* Vol. 49 (1947), pp. 5-18. Albert Tannenbaum and Herbert Silverstone: "Effect of Limited Food Intake on Survival of Mice Bearing Spontaneous Mammary Carcinoma and on the Incidence of Lung Metastases," *Cancer Research,* Vol. 13 (1953), pp. 532-6. Carlson found that intermittent fasting results in the retardation of mammary cancer in rats. Cf. Anton J. Carlson and Frederich Hoelzel: "Apparent Prolongation of the Life Span of Rats by Intermittent Fasting," *Journal of Nutrition,* Vol. 31 (1946), p. 375.

p. 15, l. 11 For the most important of these studies, see Axel Strom *et al.*: "Mortality from Circulatory Diseases in Norway, 1940-1945," *The Lancet,* Vol. 1 (1951), pp. 126-9.

p. 15, l. 31 For an excellent review of the epidemiological evidence, see Jeremiah Stammler: "The Problem of Elevated Blood Cholesterol," *American Journal of Public Health and the Nation's Health,* Vol. 50 (1960), Part II of March issue, pp. 14-19.

p. 16, l. 15 The difficulty in explaining the rising incidence of atherosclerosis and coronary heart disease is discussed exhaustively by Irvine H. Page *et al.*: "Atherosclerosis and the Fat Content of the Diet," *Circulation,* Vol. 16 (1957), pp. 163-78.

p. 17, l. 14 Alexis Carrel: *Man, the Unknown* (New York: Halcyon House; 1935), p. 39.

p. 20, l. 26 Tom Spies: "Some Recent Advances in Nutrition," *Journal of the American Medical Association,* Vol. 167 (1958), p. 690.

p. 21, l. 18   Cf. R. A. Willis: *Pathology of Tumours* (London: Butterworth & Co., Ltd.; 1953), Second Edition, p. 197.

p. 22, l. 25   Leroy E. Burney: "The Hidden Peril," *Federation Clubwoman*, Vol. 39 (1959), U. S. Public Health Service reprint; no paging.

p. 22, l. 33   Robert A. Kehoe: "Human Health and the Modern Environment," *Proceedings on "Man Versus Environment"* (Washington: U. S. Public Health Service; 1959, p. 8.

p. 24, l. 5   Surgeon General: "Environmental Health," in *Report on Environmental Health Problems: Hearings before the Subcommittee of the Committee on Appropriations, House of Representatives, 86th Congress, 2nd Session* (Washington: U. S. Government Printing Office; 1960), p. 11.

p. 24, l. 27   Ibid., pp. 6-10.

p. 27, l. 23   Wade H. Brown: "Constitutional Variation and Susceptibility to Disease," *The Harvey Lectures, 1928-1929*, Vol. 24 (Baltimore: Williams & Wilkins Company; 1930), p. 150.

p. 36, l. 6   Ralph and Mildred Buchsbaum: *Basic Ecology* (Pittsburgh: The Boxwood Press; 1957), p. 20.

Chapter Two: *Agriculture and Health*

p. 33, l. 3   Charles W. Kellogg: "We Seek; We learn," in *Soil: The Yearbook of Agriculture, 1957* (Washington: U. S. Government Printing Office), p. 4.

p. 35, l. 13   Albert Howard: *An Agricultural Testament* (London and New York: Oxford University Press; 1943), p. 1.

p. 37, l. 12   Edward Hyams: *Soil and Civilization* (London and New York: Thames and Hudson; 1952), p. 130.

p. 38, l. 34   Howard W. Lull: *Soil Compaction on Forest and Range Lands*, U. S. Department of Agriculture, Miscellaneous Publication No. 768 (Washington: U. S. Government Printing Office; 1959), p. 2.

p. 40, l. 31   A. G. Norman: "Influence of Environmental Factors on Plant Composition," *The Nutrition of Plants, Animals, and Man*, Michigan State University Centennial Symposium (1956), p. 17. Also A. G. Norman: "Soil-Plant Relationships," *American Journal of Botany*, Vol. 44 (1957), pp. 67-73.

p. 41, l. 13   Fairfield Osborn: *Our Plundered Planet* (Boston: Little, Brown & Company; 1948), pp. 68-9.

p. 42, l. 24   George L. McNew: "The Effects of Soil Fertility," in

Plant Diseases: The Yearbook of Agriculture, 1953 (Washington: U. S. Government Printing Office), p. 101.

p. 43, l. 8   Kenneth C. Beeson, statement, *Select Committee to Investigate the Use of Chemicals in Food Products, House of Representatives, 82nd Congress, 1st Session* (Washington: U. S. Government Printing Office; 1951), Part I, p. 61. Hereafter cited as *Delaney Committee Hearings.*

p. 43, l. 19   Bruce Bliven: *Preview for Tomorrow: The Unfinished Business of Science* (New York: Alfred A. Knopf, Inc.; 1953), p. 65.

p. 44, l. 14   Cf. Robert S. Harris: "The Effects of Agricultural Practices on the Composition of Foods," in *Nutritional Evaluation of Food Processing*, edited by Robert S. Harris and Harry Von Loesecke (New York and London: John Wiley & Sons, Inc.; 1960), pp. 11, 13-17.

p. 44, l. 28   For a review of the Missouri data, see William A. Albrecht: "Managing Nitrogen to Increase the Protein in Grains," *Victory Farm Forum*, Chilean Nitrate Educational Bureau, No. 43, December 1951, pp. 16-18. The Oregon and Alabama data appear in the following papers: Albert S. Hunter *et al.*: "The Effect of Nitrogen Fertilizers on the Relationship Between Increases in Yields and Protein Content of Pastry-Type Wheats," *Agronomy Journal*, Vol. 50 (1958), pp. 311-14; H. E. Sauberlich *et al.*: "The Amino Acid and Protein Content of Corn as Related to Variety and Nitrogen Fertilization," *Journal of Nutrition*, Vol. 51 (1953), pp. 241-50. Also see C. E. Evans *et al.*: "Comparisons Between Spray and Soil Applications of Nitrogen on Wheat," Research Report No. 236, U. S. Department of Agriculture, Agricultural Research Division (mimeographed; February 29, 1952), p. 56.

p. 45, l. 29   T. Lyttleton Lyon, Harry O. Buckman, and Nyle C. Brady: *The Nature and Properties of Soils* (New York: The Macmillan Company; 1952), p. 21. Also Kenneth C. Beeson: "The Effect of Fertilizers on the Nutritional Quality of Crops," *The Nutrition of Plants, Animals, and Man*, p. 47.

p. 46, l. 6   William A. Albrecht: "Soils—Their Effects on the Nutritional Values of Foods," *Consumer Bulletin*, Vol. 44 (1961), pp. 20-3. For an interesting account of the effects produced in wheat by excessive nitrogen fertilization, see K. F. Finney *et al.*: "Effects of Foliar Spraying of Pawnee Wheat with Urea Solutions on Yield, Protein Content, and Protein Quality," *Agronomy Journal*, Vol. 49 (1957), pp. 341-7. Although the foliar spraying of wheat with urea increased the protein content of the grain, Finney found that a point was eventually reached in the fertilization process where the nitrogen "produced inferior protein that possessed [bread] loaf volume potentialities equal to those usually expected from Pawnee wheat with about 1.5% less protein" (p. 345).

p. 47, l. 27   A. G. Norman: "Influence of Environmental Factors on Plant Composition," p. 17.

p. 48, l. 4   William A. Albrecht: "Our Teeth and Our Soils," *Annals of Dentistry*, Vol. 6 (1947), p. 208.

p. 48, l. 18   Kenneth C. Beeson: "Effects of the Supply of Mineral Nutrients in the Soil on the Nutritional Quality of Grasses," in *Grasslands*, edited by Howard B. Sprague (Washington: American Association for the Advancement of Science; 1959), Publication No. 53, p. 44.

p. 48, l. 35   Edward J. Thacker: "Effect of a Physiological Cation-Anion Imbalance on the Growth and Mineral Nutrition of Rabbits," *Journal of Nutrition*, Vol. 69 (1959), p. 28.

p. 49, l. 1   For example, Gennard Matrone *et al.*: *Effects of Phosphate Fertilization on the Nutritive Value of Soybean Forage for Sheep and Rabbits*, Technical Bulletin No. 1086, U. S. Department of Agriculture, May 1954. "A change in the nutritional quality of a specific nutrient with or without change in its quantity in the plants may be brought about by varying levels of soil fertility," the authors observe. "The nutritional quality of a nutrient may be simply defined as the percentage of a nutrient that is absorbed from the gastrointestinal tract and utilized by the animal. Needless to point out, the nutritional quality of a nutrient or a food is difficult to assess, necessitating carefully designed and controlled animal experiments. Because of these difficulties, a change in the nutritive quality of food crops is more likely to go undetected than a change in quantity. If this exists in fact, the insidious effects of a deterioration in the nutritional quality of our crops on the health and nutrition of animals subsisting on them may be more far-reaching and damaging than the reduction in yield or in content of nutrients in the plant" (p. 2).

p. 49, l. 13   Computed by the author from *Summary of Activities, 1950-1959*, Meat Inspection Division, U. S. Department of Agriculture (Washington: U. S. Government Printing Office).

p. 49, footnote   "Reproduction in Beef Cows: Effects of Energy and Protein Levels in Ration," Animal Husbandry Division, U. S. Department of Agriculture, Beltsville, Md. (mimeographed; April 1960), p. 1.

p. 51, l. 7   William A. Albrecht: "Managing Nitrogen to Increase the Protein in Grains," p. 17. The author has obtained additional evidence in support of Albrecht's viewpoint from a large Midwestern corn refiner. The data, covering the years 1930 to 1960, show a downward thirty-one-year trend. During most of the 1930's, the protein content of corn exceeded 10 per cent, and for three years was more than 11 per cent. By the 1950's, however, most of the yearly averages were less than 10 per cent and never exceeded 10.6 per cent.

p. 51, l. 18   Ibid.

p. 52, l. 7   William A. Albrecht: "Physical, Chemical and Biochemical Changes in the Soil Community," in *Man's Role in Changing the Face of the Earth,* edited by William L. Thomas, Jr., International Symposium, Wenner-Gren Foundation for Anthropological Research (Chicago: University of Chicago Press; 1956), p. 670.

p. 54, l. 12   The literature on this problem is enormous. For a compact body of data and comment on the effect of pesticides on all forms of wildlife, see *Miscellaneous Fish and Wildlife Bills: Hearings before the Committee on Marine and Fisheries, House of Representatives, 85th Congress, 2nd Session* (Washington: U. S. Government Printing Office; 1958), pp. 1-18. An excellent review of the problem appears in Lorus J. and Margery Milne: *The Balance of Nature* (New York: Alfred A. Knopf, Inc.; 1960), pp. 242-51. Also see John L. George: *The Pesticide Problem* (New York: The Conservation Foundation; 1957), mimeographed report; R. L. Rudd and R. E. Genelly: *Pesticides: Their Use and Toxicity in Relation to Wildlife,* Game Bulletin No. 7, California Fish and Game Department, Sacramento; G. J. Williams: "Insecticides and Birds," *Audubon Magazine,* Vol. 61 (1959), pp. 10-12, 35.

p. 54, l. 30   Charles S. Elton: *The Ecology of Invasions by Animals and Plants* (New York: John Wiley & Sons, Inc.; 1958), pp. 109-24.

p. 55, l. 2   Robert L. Rudd: "Pesticides: the *Real* Peril," *The Nation,* Vol. 189 (1959), p. 400.

p. 55, l. 38   Ibid.

p. 56, l. 4   A. W. A. Brown: *Insect Control by Chemicals* (New York: John Wiley & Sons, Inc.; 1951), p. 735.

p. 56, l. 17   Howard Baker: "Spider Mites, Insects and DDT," in *Insects: The Yearbook of Agriculture, 1952* (Washington: U. S. Government Printing Office), pp. 565, 562.

p. 57, l. 3   Edward H. Graham: "Wildlife in the Small Woodland," in *Trees: The Yearbook of Agriculture, 1949* (Washington: U. S. Government Printing Office), p. 563.

p. 57, l. 17   George J. Wallace *et al.: Bird Mortality in the Dutch*

Elm Disease Program (Bloomfield Hills, Mich.: Cranbrook Institute of Science; 1961), Bulletin No. 41, p. 10.

p. 57, l. 33 The National Audubon Society: *The Hazards of Broadcasting Toxic Pesticides* (New York: National Audubon Society; 1958), mimeographed report, p. 3.

p. 58, l. 27 Clarence Cottam: "Pesticides and Water Pollution," *Proceedings of the National Conference on Water Pollution* (Washington: U. S. Government Printing Office; 1961), p. 228. For additional data on the effects of pesticides on fish, see the series of papers in *Biological Problems in Water Pollution, Transactions of the 1959 Seminar*, The Robert A. Taft Sanitary Engineering Center, Technical Report W60-3, pp. 42-105. Also Clarence M. Tarzwell: "Pollutional Effects of Organic Insecticides," *Transactions of the Twenty-fourth North American Wildlife Conference, March 2, 3, and 4, 1959*, pp. 133-42.

p. 59, l. 12 A. W. A. Brown: *Insect Control by Chemicals*, p. 723.

p. 60, l. 20 Robert L. Rudd: "Pesticides: the *Real* Peril," p. 401.

p. 61, l. 12 William A. Albrecht: "Insoluble—Yet Available" (mimeographed paper), University of Missouri, College of Agriculture, Department of Soils, 1960, pp. 17-24.

p. 61, l. 21 Charles S. Elton: *The Ecology of Invasions by Animals and Plants*, p. 151.

Chapter Three: Urban Life and Health

p. 64, l. 13 Lewis Mumford: *The Culture of Cities* (New York: Harcourt, Brace & Company; 1938), p. 44. Also G. G. Coulton: *Medieval Panorama* (New York: The Macmillan Company; 1947), pp. 297-8.

p. 64, l. 31 Lewis Mumford: *The Culture of Cities*, p. 44.

p. 65, l. 3 Ibid., p. 50.

p. 66, l. 15 An excellent analysis of the modern work routine and its effect on the worker appears in Daniel Bell: *Work and Its Discontents* (Boston: Beacon Press; 1956), pp. 14-21.

p. 70, l. 7 This was due in large part to the work of the great American physiologist Walter B. Cannon (1871-1945). Cf. Walter B. Cannon: *Bodily Changes in Pain, Hunger, Fear and Rage* (New York and London: D. Appleton & Company; 1915).

p. 70, l. 22 It should be noted that Strümpell was still struggling with this etiological approach as recently as 1902. "In general, the disease [gastric ulcers] seems to be more frequent in the female sex than in the male; but if we count only the absolutely demonstrated cases, the difference is not a very great one. The view that ulcer of the stomach attacks by preference anemic and chlorotic girls is very general, but to the author seems much exaggerated." Adolph Strümpell: *A Text-Book of Medicine* (New York: D. Appleton & Company; 1902), Third American Edition, pp. 433-4.

p. 70, l. 34   U. S. Public Health Service: *Health Statistics from the U. S. National Health Survey, Peptic Ulcers,* Series B: No. 17, pp. 4-9. See also Table 1, p. 11. For data on the number of lives claimed by the disease, see U. S. Department of Commerce: *Statistical Abstract of the United States, 1960* (Washington: U. S. Government Printing Office), Table No. 71, p. 65.

p. 71, l. 6   National Heart Institute: *Highlights of Heart Progress, 1959* (Washington: U. S. Government Printing Office), p. 1.

p. 71, l. 25   Meyer Friedman *et al.:* "Changes in the Serum Cholesterol and Blood Clotting Time in Men Subjected to Cyclic Variation of Occupational Stress," *Circulation,* Vol. 17 (1958), p. 852. For a more generalized study of stress and serum cholesterol levels, see Meyer Friedman and R. H. Rosenman: "Association of Specific Overt Behaviour Pattern with Blood and Cardiovascular Findings," *Journal of the American Medical Association,* Vol. 169 (1959), pp. 1286-96.

p. 71, l. 34   P. T. Wertlake: "Relationship of Mental and Emotional Stress to Serum Cholesterol Levels," *New Physician,* Vol. 8 (1959), pp. 41-3, 74. See also Caroline Bedell Thomas and Edmond A. Murphy: "Further Studies on Cholesterol Levels in Johns Hopkins Medical Students: The Effect of Stress at Examinations," *Journal of Chronic Diseases,* Vol. 8 (1958), pp. 661-8.

p. 73, l. 12   Leon Hellman: "Relation of Life Stress to Arthritis," in *Life Stress and Bodily Disease,* Association for Research in Nervous and Mental Diseases, Proc. 29 (1950), p. 415.

p. 74, l. 1   Hans Selye: *The Stress of Life* (New York: McGraw-Hill Book Company, Inc., 1956), p. 131.

p. 74, l. 4   Ibid., p. 274.

p. 76, l. 21   Ibid., p. 276-7.

p. 77, l. 10   P. C. Constantinides and Niall Carey: "The Alarm Reaction," in *Scientific American Reader* (New York: Simon & Schuster; 1953), pp. 401-2.

p. 78, l. 1   Herman E. Hilleboe, statement, *Report on Environmental Health Problems,* pp. 61-3.

p. 79, l. 16   W. P. D. Logan: "Mortality in the London Fog Incident, 1952," *The Lancet,* Vol. 1 (1953), p. 337. See also Committee on Air Pollution: *Interim Report* (London: Her Majesty's Stationery Office; 1959), Cmd. 9011, pp. 16-17.

p. 80, l. 6   Harry Heimann: "Effect of Air Pollution on Human Health," in *Air Pollution,* World Health Organization (New York: Columbia University Press; 1961), p. 182.

p. 80, l. 26   New York State Air Pollution Control Board: *A Review of Air Pollution in New York State* (Albany, N.Y.; July 1958), p. 9.

p. 80, l. 31   Texas State Department of Health: *An Appraisal of Air Pollution in Texas* (Austin, Tex.; 1958), p. 1.

p. 81, l. 1   Leslie A. Chambers *et al.:* "A Comparison of Particulate Loadings in the Atmosphere of Certain American Cities," *Proceedings of the Third National Air Pollution Symposium, April 18, 19, and 20, 1955,* pp. 25-9. Herbert E. Stokinger: "Toxicologic Interaction of Air Pollutants," *International Journal of Air Pollution,* Vol. 2 (1960), pp. 321-2.

p. 81, l. 25   John H. Ludwig: "Some Ramifications of Air Contamination," *Public Health Reports,* Vol. 75 (1960), p. 413.

p. 82, l. 8   Leslie A. Chambers: "Where Does Air Pollution Come From?" *Proceedings of the National Conference on Air Pollution,* op. cit., pp. 35-7.

p. 83, l. 10   "The mechanism is not clear, but may represent a binding of carbon monoxide by the tissues chronically exposed to it, particularly muscle myoglobin, which has a strong affinity for the gas, and the nervous system, from which it is then slowly released into the blood." Gordon J. Gilbert and Gilbert H. Glaser: "Neurologic Manifestations of Chronic Carbon Monoxide Poisoning," *New England Journal of Medicine,* Vol. 261 (1958), p. 1219.

p. 83, l. 17   Richard Prindle: *The Disaster Potential of Community Air Pollution,* U. S. Public Health Service (mimeographed; no paging), January 1960. This paper has recently been published in *The Air We Breathe,* edited by Farber and Wilson (Springfield, Ill.: Charles C Thomas; 1961). See also John R. Goldsmith and Lewis H. Rogers: "Health Hazards of Automobile Exhaust," *Public Health Reports,* Vol. 74 (1959), pp. 553-4.

p. 84, l. 1   Gorden E. McCallum and John R. Thomas: "Sewage Treatment Needs of the United States," *Sewage and Industrial Wastes,* Vol. 31 (1959), pp. 3-5. Also Task Group 2450R Report: "Survey of Ground Water Contamination and Waste Disposal Practices," *American Water Works Association, Journal,* Vol. 52 (1960), pp. 1211-19.

p. 84, l. 15 Graham Walton: *ABS Contamination of Water Resources,* The Robert A. Taft Sanitary Engineering Center (mimeographed; April 1960), pp. 5-10. Richard L. Woodward: *Pesticides and Water Supplies,* The Robert A. Taft Sanitary Engineering Center (mimeographed; April 1960), pp. 4-5. A. R. Todd: "Water Purification Upset Seriously by Detergents," *Water and Sewage Works,* Vol. 101 (1954). p. 80. Lloyd R. Setter *et al.:* "Radioactivity of Surface Waters in the United States," *American Water Works Association, Journal,* Vol. 51 (1959), pp. 1387-9. Ernest A. Snow: "Radioactive Fallout and Drinking Water," *New England Water Works Association, Journal,* Vol. 75 (1961), pp. 27-37.

p. 84, l. 21 Rolf Eliassen: "Research and Treatment Technology," *Proceedings of the National Conference on Water Pollution,* p. 456.

p. 85, l. 1 T. A. Filipi, Nebraska State Department of Public Health, quoted by Alvin B. Toffler: "Danger in Your Drinking Water," *Good Housekeeping,* January 1960, p. 129.

p. 85, l. 14 Norman A. Clarke and Shih Lu Chang: "Enteric Viruses in Water," *American Water Works Association, Journal,* Vol. 51 (1959), pp. 1300-3.

p. 87, l. 3 Rene Dubos: *The Mirage of Health* (New York: Harper & Brothers; 1959), p. 172.

p. 87, l. 17 Richard A. Prindle: *The Disaster Potential of Community Air Pollution.* Also I. J. Brightman: *Air Pollution and Health: New Facts from New York State,* New York State Air Pollution Control Board (mimeographed; June 1961), pp. 5-9.

Chapter Four: The Problem of Chemicals in Food

p. 89, l. 9 Allen B. Paul and Lorenzo B. Mann: "What Our Grandparents Did Not Have," in *Marketing: The Yearbook of Agriculture, 1954* (Washington: U. S. Government Printing Office), p. 121.

p. 91, l. 3 R. C. Burrell *et al.:* "Ascorbic Acid Content of Cabbage as Influenced by Variety, Season and Soil Fertilizers," *Food Research,* Vol. 5 (1940), pp. 247-52. H. B. N. Murthy and M. Swaminathan: "The Nutritive Value of Different Varieties of Sweet Potato," *Current Science,* Vol. 23 (1954), Letter to Editor, p. 14. Paul R. Burkholder *et al.:* "Niacin in Maize," *Yale Journal of Biological Medicine,* Vol. 16 (1944), pp. 659-63.

p. 91, l. 9 Henry C. Sherman: *Chemistry of Food and Nutrition*

(New York: The Macmillan Company; 1952), Eighth Edition, p. 621.

p. 91, l. 14   Cf. Robert S. Harris: "The Effects of Agricultural Practices on the Composition of Foods," in *Nutritional Evaluation of Food Processing,* pp. 22-3.

p. 91, footnote   Ibid., p. 6.

p. 92, l. 4   Cf. E. J. Cameron *et al.:* "Nutrient Retention during Canned Food Production," *American Journal of Public Health and the Nation's Health,* Vol. 39 (1949), pp. 756-63.

p. 92, l. 7   Mildred M. Boggs and Clyde L. Rasmussen: "Modern Food Processing," in *Food: The Yearbook of Agriculture, 1959* (Washington: U. S. Government Printing Office), p. 420.

p. 92, l. 14   L. Jean Bogert: *Nutrition and Physical Fitness,* p. 232. Also Samuel Lepkovsky: "The Bread Problem in War and in Peace," *Physiological Reviews,* Vol. 24 (1944) pp. 239-76. H. M. Sinclair: "The Composition and Nutritive Value of Flour," *Royal Society of Health, Journal,* Vol. 77 (1957), pp. 235-42.

p. 92, l. 21   Bernice Kunerth Watt and Woot-Tsuen Wu Leung: "Conserving Nutritive Values," in *Food: The Yearbook of Agriculture, 1959,* p. 486.

p. 92, l. 34   Jesse V. Coles: "Compulsory Grade Labeling," in *Marketing: The Yearbook of Agriculture, 1954* (Washington: U. S. Government Printing Office), p. 168.

p. 93, l. 19   For a number of choice examples, see Select Committee to Investigate the Use of Chemicals in Food Products: *Report No. 2356, House of Representatives, 82nd Congress, 2nd Session* (Washington: U. S. Government Printing Office; June 30, 1952), pp. 4-12, 17-20.

p. 94, l. 2   Franklin Bicknell: *Chemicals in Your Food and in Farm Produce: Their Harmful Effects* (New York: Emerson Books, Inc.; 1961). Also B. S. Platt: "Human Nutrition and the Sophistication of Foods and Feeding Habits," *British Medical Journal,* Vol. 1 (1955), pp. 180-1.

p. 94, footnote   Cf. OPD Reports from Europe: "Unilever Food Additive 'Episode' Is Running Up a Tab of $2 Million," *Oil, Paint and Drug Reporter,* May 22, 1961, p. 5.

p. 95, l. 10   Consumers' Union: "Chemicals in Our Food Supply," *Consumer Reports,* Vol. 21 (1956), p. 456.

p. 96, l. 4   Compare Roy C. Newton, statement, *Delaney Committee Hearings,* 1950, pp. 156-60, and John Foulger, statement, ibid., pp. 505-8.

p. 97, l. 4   George C. Decker, statement, *Delaney Committee Hearings,* Part I, p. 179.

p. 97, l. 22   A. W. A. Brown: *Insect Control by Chemicals*, p. 721.

p. 98, l. 21   Arthur Kallet and F. J. Schlink: *100,000,000 Guinea Pigs* (New York: Grosset & Dunlap; 1933), pp. 50-1.

p. 98, l. 32   A. W. A. Brown: *Insect Control by Chemicals*, pp. 548-9. For data on the accumulation of organic insecticides in the soil, see Robert D. Chisholm and Louis Koblitsky: "Accumulation and Dissipation of Pesticide Residues in Soil," *Transactions of the Twenty-fourth North American Wildlife Conference, March 2, 3, and 4, 1959*, pp. 119-23.

p. 99, l. 10   Lucille F. Stickel and Paul F. Springer: *Pesticides and Wildlife*, U. S. Fish and Wildlife Service, Wildlife Leaflet 392 (no date), p. 1.

p. 100, l. 6   For a succinct review of theories on the toxic activity of DDT, see Robert L. Metcalf: *The Mode of Action of Organic Insecticides* (Washington: National Research Council; 1948), pp. 52-5. See also Council on Pharmacy and Chemistry: "Pharmacologic and Toxicologic Aspects of DDT (Chlorophenothane, U.S.P.)," *Journal of the American Medical Association*, Vol. 145 (1951), pp. 728-33.

p. 100, footnote   S. Gershon and F. H. Shaw: "Psychiatric Sequelae of Chronic Exposure to Organophosphorus Insecticides," *The Lancet*, Vol. 1 (1961), pp. 1371-4.

p. 101, l. 21   A. J. Lehman: "Conservatism in Estimating the Hazards of Pesticidal Residues," *Association of Food and Drug Officials of the United States, Quarterly Bulletin*, Vol. 18 (1954), p. 88. Also Paul Ortega *et al.*: *DDT in the Diet of the Rat*, U. S. Public Health Service, Public Health Monograph No. 43 (Washington: U. S. Government Printing Office; 1956), p. 18.

p. 101, l. 24   The following comment by Emil M. Mrak before the 1960 Joint Conference of the F.D.A. and the Food Law Institute seems to speak for itself: "It was also apparent that one of the factors involved in the problem [of DDT residues in dairy products] was the existence of a tolerance of 7 p.p.m. for DDT on hay produced in California. When this tolerance was set, it was not generally known that the halogenated hydrocarbons would be concentrated in the fat of milk. It is well known now, however, that when a cow feed is contaminated with DDT or related compounds, the material will be concentrated in the fat and when milk is converted to butter or evaporated milk, the agricultural chemical concentrates accordingly." Emil M. Mrak: "Public Awareness of Health Aspects of Chemical Aids," *Food, Drug, Cosmetic Law Journal*, Vol. 16 (1961), pp. 18-19.

p. 101, l. 31   Quoted by *The New York Times*, December 15, 1959.

p. 102, l. 4   W. N. Bruce: "Insecticides and Flies," in *Insects: The Yearbook of Agriculture, 1952*, p. 321.

p. 102, l. 16   Select Committee to Investigate the Use of Chemicals in Food Products: *Report No. 2356*, p. 14.

p. 102, l. 24   Cf. W. I. Patterson and A. J. Lehman: "Pesticides: Some Chemical Considerations and Toxicological Interpretations," *Association of Food and Drug Officials of the United States, Quarterly Bulletin*, Vol. 17 (1953), Table II, p. 11.

p. 102, l. 29   A. J. Lehman: "Some Toxicological Reasons Why Certain Chemicals May or May Not Be Permitted as Food Additives," *Association of Food and Drug Officials of the United States, Quarterly Bulletin*, Vol. 14 (1950), pp. 92-3.

p. 103, l. 10   A. J. Lehman: "Conservatism in Estimating the Hazards of Pesticidal Residues," p. 90.

p. 103, l. 25   Herbert F. Schoof: "Recent Developments in Pesticides," *American Journal of Public Health and the Nation's Health*, Vol. 50 (1960), p. 632.

p. 104, l. 1   Agricultural Chemicals Staff: *The Pesticide Situation for 1959-1960*, U. S. Department of Agriculture, Food and Materials Division, Washington, April 1960, p. 3. See previous issues of this annual report for long-range statistical data on the output of pesticides.

p. 104, l. 3   Clarence Cottam: "Pesticides and Water Pollution," p. 223.

p. 104, l. 27   Select Committee to Investigate the Use of Chemicals in Food Products: *Report No. 2356*, p. 10.

p. 104, l. 34   R. W. Detwiler *et al.:* "The Influence of Thiouracil and Stilbestrol on Broiler Quality," *Poultry Science*, Vol. 29 (1950), pp. 513-19. Detwiler observes that "all lots on experimental treatment contained significantly greater quantities of fat and less protein and moisture than the controls" (p. 515). See also T. C. Byerly: "Hormone in Feeds," in *Symposium on Medicated Feeds*, edited by Henry Welch and Félix Martí-Ibáñez (New York: Medical Encyclopedia, Inc.; 1956), p. 17. According to Byerly, the breast-muscle fat content of chickens is doubled.

p. 105, l. 3   R. K. Enders, testimony, *Delaney Committee Hearings*, Part I, p. 432.

p. 105, l. 20   U. S. Food and Drug Administration: *Chronology Relating to the Use of Diethylstilbestrol in Poultry and Meat Animals* (mimeographed; December 1959), p. 4.

p. 106, l. 12   William A. Randall: "Antibiotic Residues," in *First International Conference on Antibiotics in Agriculture* (Washington: National Academy of Sciences-National Research Council; 1956), p. 261.

p. 107, l. 1 The following comment by an Indiana food-control official gives a vivid idea of the difficulties involved in controlling spray residues in food: "Without prior knowledge of its application, there will be a great deal of difficulty to determine what pesticide or spray residue the laboratory should look for in a given sample of a raw agricultural product. Approximately 3,000 tolerances have been set for over 200 pesticides ranging all the way from Aldrin to Ziram. In order for the laboratory to test a submitted sample, it is necessary for that laboratory to know what pesticide has been or may have been used. This, in turn, means that a great deal of field work must be instituted so prior knowledge may be obtained. It means that field men from the state agency must visit the producing farms, greenhouses, or orchards, and determine what is being used, when, and how much. Although the pesticide manufacturer is required to label his products with adequate directions for use, including information as to which crop it is to be used on, and when, and in what quantity, there is no valid assurance that the agriculturists will use it according to directions or limit it to the crops on which it safely may be used. It becomes necessary for the field man to determine, insofar as possible, what insecticide the agriculturist is using, on which crop, and what prohibited insecticide may have been used. All this must be done during the growing season, but samples of the finished agricultural products cannot be obtained until the time of harvest or after shipment. Where a violation is suspected, the sampling of the mature raw agricultural commodity must be prompt or the product will have been shipped, distributed, and consumed." T. E. Sullivan: "Spray Residues on Fruits and Vegetables," *Journal of Milk and Food Technology*, Vol. 24 (1961), p. 154.

p. 107, l. 8 Letter from Arthur S. Flemming to Rep. Oren Harris, April 18, 1960, reproduced in *Color Additives; Hearings before the Committee on Interstate and Foreign Commerce, House of Representatives, 86th Congress, 2nd Session* (Washington: U. S. Government Printing Office; 1960), p. 218.

p. 107, l. 32 Murray C. Zimmerman: "Chronic Penicillin Urticaria from Dairy Products Proved by Penicillinase Cures," *A.M.A. Archives of Dermatology*, Vol. 79 (1959), pp. 2-3. See also H. R. Vickers *et al.*: "Dermatitis Caused by Penicillin in Milk," *The Lancet*, Vol. 1 (1958), p. 351.

p. 108, l. 19 H. William Smith: "Drug-Resistant Bacteria in Domestic Animals," *Proceedings of the Royal Society of Medicine*, Vol. 51 (1958), p. 813.

p. 109, l. 4 Ibid., p. 812.

p. 109, l. 9 F. S. Thatcher and W. Simon: "The Resistance of Staphylococci and Streptococci Isolated from Cheese to Various Antibiotics," *Canadian Journal of Public Health*, Vol. 46 (1955), p. 409.

p. 110, l. 1 Joseph S. Pagano et al.: "Isolation from Animals of Human Strains of Staphylococci during an Epidemic in a Veterinary School," *Science*, Vol. 131 (1960), pp. 927-8. The term "human strains of staphylococci" may be misleading. "There is not a clearly defined demarcation between human and animal strains of *Staphylococcus aureus*," note Zinn, Anderson, and Skaggs, "even though these terms are frequently used. . . . A human 'epidemic' strain of *Staph. aureus* has produced persistent furunculosis in a herd of dairy cows attended by persons harboring such staphylococci in their anterior nares. The bovine species may thus serve as an additional host for antibiotic-resistant staphylococci which are currently a major problem in human hospitals." Raymond D. Zinn et al.: "Staphylococci Infection in Cattle," *Journal of the American Veterinary Medical Association*, Vol. 138 (1961), p. 386. See also Gorden D. Wallace et al.: "Preliminary Report of Human Staphylococcal Infection Associated with Mastitis in Dairy Cattle," *Public Health Reports*, Vol. 75 (1960), pp. 457-60.

p. 110, l. 32. Cf. Daniel McKinley: "Nature and Man: The Two Faces of Management," *Audubon Magazine*, Vol. 62 (1960), pp. 104-6, 138-9, 144.

p. 111, l. 12 Robert M. Ikeda and Donald G. Crosby: *Chemicals and the Food Industry* (Berkeley: University of California, Division of Agricultural Sciences; 1960), p. 33.

p. 112, l. 10 Anton J. Carlson, testimony, *Delaney Committee Hearings*, 1950, p. 8.

p. 112, l. 21 Quoted by *The New York Times*, May 19, 1953.

p. 112, l. 22 Cf. Edward Eagle, statement, *Delaney Committee Hearings*, 1950, pp. 297-305.

p. 112, l. 29 Cf. C. E. Poling et al.: "Effects of Feeding Polyoxyethylene Preparations to Rats and Hamsters," *Food Research*, Vol. 21 (1956), pp. 337-47.

p. 112, footnote (l. 2) Unpublished reports by the Food and Drug Administration, described and cited in *The Safety of Polyoxyethylene* (8) *Stearate for Use in Food*, Food Protection

Committee, Food and Nutrition Board (Washington: National Academy of Sciences–National Research Council; December 1958), Publication 646, pp. 8-9.

p. 113, l. 5   F. J. Schlink, statement, *Delaney Committee Hearings*, 1950, p. 743.

p. 113, footnote (l. 1)   W. C. Hueper: "Potential Cancer Hazards from Cosmetics to Producers and Consumers," *Drug Research Reports*, September 28, 1960, pp. 440-S-441-S.

p. 114, l. 9   Cf. Oscar E. Anderson, Jr.: *The Health of a Nation: Harvey Wiley and the Fight for Pure Food* (Chicago: University of Chicago Press; 1958), p. 215.

p. 114, l. 14   Mrs. Harvey Wiley, testimony, *Delaney Committee Hearings*, 1950, p. 833.

p. 114, l. 21   Robert M. Ikeda and Donald G. Crosby: *Chemicals and the Food Industry*, pp. 93-127. Also Food and Drug Administration: *Compilation of Regulations for Food Additives*, U. S. Department of Health, Education, and Welfare, Subpart A—Food Additives.

p. 114, footnote   Ministry of Agriculture, Fisheries, and Food: *Food Standards Committee Report on Preservatives in Food* (London: Her Majesty's Stationery Office; 1959), Appendix IV, pp. 63-70.

p. 115, l. 24   Cf. Harry E. Goresline: "Food Spoilage and Deterioration," in *Handbook of Food and Agriculture*, edited by Fred C. Blank (New York: Reinhold Publishing Corporation; 1955), p. 406.

p. 116, l. 9   A. J. Lehman: "Nitrates and Nitrites in Meat Products," *Association of Food and Drug Officials of the United States, Quarterly Bulletin*, Vol. 22 (1958), p. 138.

p. 116, l. 23   George L. Prichard, testimony, *Delaney Committee Hearings*, 1950, p. 418.

p. 117, l. 7   Select Committee to Investigate the Use of Chemicals in Food Products: *Report No. 2356*, p. 19.

p. 117, l. 33   U. S. Food and Drug Administration: *What Consumers Should Know about Food Additives* (Washington: U. S. Government Printing Office; 1959), no paging.

p. 118, l. 27   Cf. W. C. Hueper: "The Potential Role of Non-Nutritive Food Additives and Contaminants as Environmental Carcinogens," *A.M.A. Archives of Pathology*, Vol. 62 (1956), p. 226.

p. 118, l. 29   Cf. W. Heupke: "Ernährungsschäden durch technische Bearbeitung der Lebensmittel und durch in Ernährungsindustrie verwendete Substanzen," *Osterreichische Arztezeitung*, Vol. 16, No. 10 (1961)—Print.

p. 118, l. 35   A. J. Lehman: "Conservatism in Estimating the Hazards of Pesticidal Residues," p. 89.

p. 119, l. 32   United Press International, April 10, 1961. To be published in a future issue of the *A.M.A. Archives of Pathology.*

p. 120, l. 3   Wallace F. Janssen, Food and Drug Administration (personal communication).

Chapter Five: Environment and Cancer

p. 122, l. 10   Cf. W. C. Hueper: "Age Aspects of Environmental and Occupational Cancers," *Public Health Reports,* Vol. 67 (1952), pp. 773-9.

p. 122, l. 14   Sigismund Peller: *Cancer in Man* (New York: International Universities Press; 1952), p. 45.

p. 122, l. 25   Cf. Maud Slye: "Biological Evidence for the Inheritability of Cancer in Man," *Journal of Cancer Research,* Vol. 7 (1922), pp. 107-47.

p. 122, l. 33   "The available statistical and experimental evidence shows clearly, I think, that while an inherited predisposition to particular kinds of tumours is sometimes discernible, and is in occasional special instances paramount, by far the larger number of human cancers is due to carcinogenic chemical or other stimuli which are probably effective in most adequately exposed individuals whatever their genetic inheritance." R. A. Willis: *Pathology of Tumours,* p. 91.

p. 123, l. 4   Sigismund Peller: *Cancer in Man,* p. 59.

p. 123, l. 12   Cf. Charles Oberling: *The Riddle of Cancer* (New Haven: Yale University Press; 1952), p. 83.

p. 123, l. 19   Ibid.

p. 124, l. 5   Sigismund Peller: *Cancer in Man,* p. 184.

p. 124, l. 35   Edmund G. Zimmerer and William M. Haenszel: *Cancer in Iowa,* U. S. Public Health Service, Public Health Service Publication No. 466 (Washington: U. S. Government Printing Office; 1956), p. 3. For a more detailed report of this survey, see William M. Haenszel, Samuel C. Marcus, and Edward C. Zimmerer: *Cancer Morbidity in Urban and Rural Iowa,* U. S. Public Health Service, Public Health Monograph No. 37 (Washington: U. S. Government Printing Office; 1956).

p. 125, l. 9   Harold F. Dorn and Sidney J. Cutler: *Morbidity from Cancer in the United States,* p. 106.

p. 125, l. 18   Cf. W. C. Hueper: *Environmental and Occupational Cancer,* U. S. Public Health Service, Supplement 209 to *Public Health Reports* (Washington: U. S. Government Printing Office; 1948), pp. 8, 35-47. Also see P. Stocks: "Cancer of the Uterine Cervix and Social Conditions," *British Journal of Cancer,* Vol. 9 (1955), pp. 487-94. "A study of the death-rates in 48 large towns in 1950-52," observes Stocks, shows a relationship with overcrowding, social class distribution and predominant industry 20 years before. Seaports and textile towns have high rates for cervix cancer . . ." (pp. 493-4).

p. 125, l. 29   W. C. Hueper: *Environmental and Occupational Cancer,* p. 2.

p. 126, l. 33   It should be noted that this widely used figure refers to "discovered" cases of cancer in a given year. Cutler and Haenszel, writing in 1954, estimated that over a half million new cases of cancer develop annually. It was their opinion that by 1960 the number of newly developed cancer cases would reach 605,000 a year, and by 1975, about 750,000. Cf. Sidney J. Cutler and William M. Haenszel: "The Magnitude of the Cancer Problem," *Public Health Reports,* Vol. 69 (1954), Table 1, p. 334.

p. 127, l. 7   "Evidence is accumulating that 'spontaneous' cancers are actually induced. . . . In fact, the more we learn about everything, the less use there is for 'spontaneous,' for all effects have their causes even though we cannot identify them." Editorial: "Puncturing the Spontaneous," *CA: Bulletin of Cancer Progress,* Vol. 7 (1957), No. 1.

p. 127, l. 13   Charles Oberling: *The Riddle of Cancer,* p. 86.

p. 129, l. 9   Eugene P. Pendergrass: *Annual Address* (unpublished typescript furnished by the American Cancer Society), pp. 11-12.

p. 129, l. 18   Quoted by the *New York Post,* October 27, 1959.

p. 130, l. 8   Hans Selye: *The Stress of Life,* p. 187.

p. 130, l. 21   Cf. Richard R. Howard and Wendell A. Grosjean: "Bilateral Mammary Carcinoma in the Male Coincident with Prolonged Stilbestrol Therapy," *Surgery,* Vol. 25 (1949), pp. 300-3. D. G. Corbett and Edward Abrams: "Bilateral Carcinoma of the Male Breasts Associated with Prolonged Stilbestrol for Carcinoma of the Prostate," *Journal of Urology,* Vol. 64 (1950), pp. 377-81. Corbett and Abrams note that "the fact that in this case the condition was bilateral, and also the paucity of reports of metastatic growth in the breasts of patients with carcinoma of the prostate before the wide use of stilbestrol, make it impossible for us to ignore the

relationship of hormonal therapy to these breast carcinomas"
(p. 380).
p. 130, l. 23   Charles Oberling: *The Riddle of Cancer*, p. 104.

p. 130, l. 30   Sheldon C. Sommers: "Endocrine Abnormalities in
Women with Breast Cancer," *Laboratory Investigation*, Vol. 4
(1955), pp. 160-74.

p. 131, l. 6   Cf. Raymond F. Kaiser: "Possible Diagnostic Implications in Cancer Research," *CA: Bulletin of Cancer Progress*,
Vol. 11 (1961), pp. 10-11.

p. 131, p. 13   Eugene P. Pendergrass: *Annual Address*, p. 12.
For a criticism of professional indifference to the relationship
between stress and cancer, see E. M. Blumberg *et al.*: "A Pos-
sible Relationship Between Psychological Factors and Human
Cancer," *Psychosomatic Medicine*, Vol. 16 (1954), p. 285.
See also L. LeShan: "Psychological States as Factors in the
Development of Malignant Disease," *Journal of the National
Cancer Institute*, Vol. 22 (1959), pp. 1-18. G. M. Perrin and
I. R. Pierce: "Psychosomatic Aspects of Cancer," *Psychoso-
matic Medicine*, Vol. 21 (1959), pp. 397-421.

p. 132, l. 6   Charles Oberling: *The Riddle of Cancer*, p. 196.

p. 132, l. 18   Sloan-Kettering Institute for Cancer Research:
Progress Report XI, New York (1958), pp. 14-15.

p. 133, l. 3   "Liver Cancer in Bantu and American Negro," *Nutrition Reviews*, Vol. 3 (1945), pp. 19-21. For an excellent review article on nutrition and cancer, see H. P. Rusch and
C. A. Baumann: "Nutritional Aspects of Cancer Problem,"
Nutrition Reviews, Vol. 4 (1946), pp. 353-5.

p. 133, l. 9   Sigismund Peller: *Cancer in Man*, p. 255.

p. 133, l. 15   Helen N. Lovell: "Diet in Cancer," *Journal of the
Iowa State Medical Society*, Vol. 39 (1949), p. 295.

p. 136, l. 3   Sigismund Peller: *Cancer in Man*, p. 114. Peller's
work contains a superb historical review of research on environmental cancer. See also R. E. Eckardt: *Industrial Carcinogens* (New York and London: Grune and Stratton; 1959),
pp. 1-12, 14-23.

p. 136, l. 31   W. C. Hueper *et al.*: "Experimental Induction of
Bladder Tumors in Dogs by Administration of Beta-Naphthalamine," *Journal of Industrial Hygiene and Toxicology*, Vol.
20 (1938), pp. 46-84.

p. 137, l. 2   Subcommittee on Carcinogenesis (Food Protection
Committee): *Problems in the Evaluation of Carcinogenic
Hazards from the Use of Food Additives* (Washington: National Academy of Sciences–National Research Council;
1959), Publication 749, p. 21. For a vigorous criticism of the
light-minded recommendations made by this subcommittee,

see the testimony of Harold L. Stewart, of the National Cancer Institute, in *Color Additives*, pp. 410-19, 428-33.

p. 137, l. 22   W. C. Hueper: "The Potential Role of Non-Nutritive Food Additives and Contaminants as Environmental Carcinogens," p. 226.

p. 138, l. 3   However, adenocarcinoma of the stomach has finally been produced in rats by feeding the animals N,N'-2,7-Fluorenylenebisacetamide. Although a chemical carcinogen has now been found that produces this type of stomach cancer in rats by means of feeding experiments, the disease has not been produced by feeding rats carcinogens that are suspected of causing adenocarcinoma of the stomach in man. Cf. Harold L. Stewart *et al.*: "Carcinoma of the Glandular Stomach of Rats Ingesting N,N'2,7-Fluorenylenebisacetamide," *National Cancer Institute Monograph No. 5* (1961), p. 106.

p. 138, l. 7   Robert E. Eckardt: *Industrial Carcinogens*, p. 60.

p. 138, l. 17   Recommendations for carcinogenicity tests of food additives vary widely from one country to another. Cf. Bernard L. Oser's discussion in "The Scientists' Forum" of the *Food, Drug, Cosmetic Law Journal*, Vol. 16 (1961), pp. 290-1.

p. 139, l. 3   Food Protection Committee (Food and Nutrition Board): *The Use of Chemical Additives in Food Processing* (Washington: National Academy of Sciences–National Research Council; February 1956), Publication 398, pp. 31, 79, 43, 55-6.

p. 139, l. 14   Walter D. Conway and Elizabeth Lethco: "Aromatic Amine Impurities in Yellow AB and Yellow OB Food Dyes," *Analytic Chemistry*, Vol. 32 (1960), pp. 838-41.

p. 139, l. 30   Francis E. Ray, testimony, *Delaney Committee Hearings*, 1950, p. 641.

p. 140, l. 13   U. S. Food and Drug Administration: *Chronology Relating to the Use of Diethylstilbestrol in Poultry and Meat Animals*, p. 3.

p. 140, l. 31   F. O. Gossett *et al.*: "The Feeding of High Levels of Diethylstilbestrol to Beef Steers," in *Symposium on Medicated Feeds*, p. 97. Charles W. Turner: "Biological Assay of Beef Steer Carcasses for Estrogenic Activity Following the Feeding of Diethylstilbestrol at a Level of 10 Mg. per Day in the Ration," *Journal of Animal Science*, Vol. 15 (1956), p. 19.

p. 140, footnote   Cf. W. C. Hueper: "Potential Cancer Hazards from Cosmetics to Producers and Consumers," pp. 439-s-440-s.

p. 141, l. 6   H. B. Andervont *et al.*: "Some Factors Involved in the Induction or Growth of Testicular Tumors in BALB/c Mice," *Journal of the National Cancer Institute* (in press).

p. 141, l. 17   G. Hadfield: "Co-carcinogenesis," *Proceedings of the Royal Society of Medicine*, Vol. 49 (1956), pp. 662-4.

p. 141, l. 21   Paul E. Steiner and Hans L. Falk: "Summation and Inhibition Effects of Weak and Strong Carcinogenic Hydrocarbons: 1:2-Benzanthracene, Chrysene, 1:2:5:6-Dibenzanthracene, and 20-Methylcholanthrene," *Cancer Research*, Vol. 10 (1951), pp. 56-63.

p. 141, l. 26   W. C. Hueper: "The Potential Role of Non-Nutritive Food Additives and Contaminants as Environmental Carcinogens," p. 226.

p. 142, l. 9   Harold L. Stewart, testimony, *Color Additives*, pp. 418-19.

p. 142, l. 11   Cf. M. M. Hargraves: "Chemical Pesticides and Conservation Problems," *Twenty-third Annual Convention of the National Wildlife Federation* (mimeographed; February 27, 1959), pp. 3-4.

p. 142, l. 17   Hans Falk *et al.*: "Milk as an Eluant of Polycyclic Aromatic Hydrocarbons Added to Wax," *Nature*, Vol. 183 (1959), p. 1184.

p. 142, l. 22   Hueper, in fact, concludes from the evidence at hand that crude and semi-refined paraffins and waxes "possess definite carcinogenic properties to man and animals . . ." W. C. Hueper: "Potential Cancer Hazards from Cosmetics to Producers and Consumers," p. 437-S.

p. 142, l. 28   J. W. Cook: "Chemical Carcinogens and Their Significance," *The Lancet*, Vol. 1 (1957), pp. 333-5.

p. 143, l. 2   Paul Kotin: "Experimentally Weak Carcinogens," *Cancer Research*, Vol. 18 (1958), p. 3.

p. 143, l. 18   Sigismund Peller: *Cancer in Man*, p. 6.

p. 144, l. 5   E. Cuyler Hammond: "Smoking and Death Rates— A Riddle in Cause and Effect," *American Scientist*, Vol. 46 (1958), p. 331.

p. 144, l. 9   Jerome Cornfield *et al.*: "Smoking and Lung Cancer," *Journal of the National Cancer Institute*, Vol. 22 (1959), p. 176.

p. 144, l. 17   Ibid., p. 177.

p. 144, l. 33   Ibid., p. 176.

p. 145, l. 24   E. C. Hammond: "Cigarette Smoking and Disease," *American Biology Teacher*, Vol. 21 (1959), pp. 289-90.

p. 146, l. 31   Cf. E. Cuyler Hammond and Daniel Horn: "Smoking and Death Rates—Report on Forty-four Months of Follow-up of 187,783 Men," *Journal of the American Medical Association*, Vol. 166 (1958), pp. 1159-72, 1294-1308.

p. 147, l. 12   Oscar Auerbach *et al.*: "Changes in Bronchial Epithelium in Relation to Cigarette Smoking and in Relation to Lung Cancer," *New England Journal of Medicine,* Vol. 295 (1961), pp. 253-67.

p. 148, l. 25   Cf. Geoffrey Dean: "Lung Cancer Among White South Africans," *British Medical Journal,* Vol. 2 (1959), pp. 852-7.

p. 149, l. 12   E. L. Wynder *et al.*: "Dose-Response Studies with Benzo[a]pyrene," *Cancer,* Vol. 13 (1960), pp. 106-10.

p. 149, l. 15   Eugene Sawicki *et al.*: *Benzo[a]pyrene Content of the Air of American Communities,* The Robert A. Taft Sanitary Engineering Center (mimeographed; no date), Table VII.

p. 149, l. 25   W. C. Hueper *et al.*: *Carcinogenic Bioassays on Air Pollutants,* U. S. Public Health Service (mimeographed; 1960), Table 1.

p. 149, l. 28:   For a good review of Kotin's data and their significance, see W. C. Hueper: *A Quest into the Environmental Causes of Cancer of the Lung,* U. S. Public Health Service, Public Health Monograph No. 36 (Washington: U. S. Government Printing Office; 1955), pp. 6-8.

p. 151, l. 3   Fritz Lickint: "Tabak und Tabakrauch als ätiologischer Factor des Carcinoms," *Zeitschrift für Krebsforschung,* Vol. 30 (1929-30), pp. 349-65.

p. 151, l. 6   William D. McNally: "The Tar in Cigarette Smoke and Its Possible Effects," *American Journal of Cancer,* Vol. 16 (1932), pp. 1511-12.

p. 151, l. 8   Alton Ochsner and Michael DeBakey: "Carcinoma of the Lung," *Archives of Surgery,* Vol. 42 (1941), pp. 219-21. One of the most interesting features of this early paper is the discussion presented by the authors on the rising incidence of lung cancer (pp. 209-14).

p. 152, l. 6   Quoted by *The New York Times,* May 19, 1961.

p. 152, l. 19   Lester Breslow: *Air Pollution and Cancer,* Fourth National Cancer Conference (paper unpublished at this writing).

Chapter Six: *Radiation and Human Health*

p. 154, l. 9   Samuel G. Ingraham *et al.*: *Concepts of Radiological Health,* U. S. Public Health Service, Public Health Service Publication No. 336 (Washington; January 1954), p. 2.

p. 155, l. 9   Jack Schubert and Ralph Lapp: *Radiation: What It Is and How It Affects You* (New York: The Viking Press; 1957), p. 124. Also see Robert D. Evans and Robert A. Dudley: "The Radium 226 Standard for Bone Seekers," in

Selected Materials on Radiation Protection Criteria and Standards: Their Basis and Use, Joint Committee on Atomic Energy, Congress of the United States, 86th Congress, 2nd Session (Washington: U. S. Government Printing Office; 1960), p. 438.

p. 155, l. 23   W. F. Neuman: "The Somatic Effects of Fission Products," *Bulletin of the Atomic Scientists*, Vol. 14 (1958), p. 17. Schubert and Lapp, however, give strontium-90 one fifth the toxicity of radium. "Our reason for reducing the permissible level of strontium-90 is that more recent experiments (by Dr. Miriam P. Finkel of the Argonne National Laboratory) on the induction of bone tumors in mice have shown that strontium-90 is indeed more toxic than previously thought." Jack Schubert and Ralph Lapp: *Radiation: What It Is and How It Affects You*, p. 127.

p. 160, l. 7   Hugh F. Henry: *Is All Nuclear Radiation Harmful?* A.E.C. Research and Development Report, K-1470 (mimeographed; May 2, 1961), pp. 12-13.

p. 160, l. 27   John T. Gentry *et al.*: "An Epidemiological Study of Congenital Malformation in New York State," *American Journal of Public Health and the Nation's Health*, Vol. 49 (1959), pp. 497-513. For a statistical evaluation of the significance of Gentry's data, see James E. McDonald: "A Study in Genetic Damage," in *Fallout from Nuclear Weapons Tests: Hearings before the Special Subcommittee on Radiation of the Joint Committee on Atomic Energy, Congress of the United States, 86th Congress, 1st Session* (Washington: U. S. Government Printing Office; 1959), Vol. 3, pp. 2402-22; hereafter cited as *JCAE, 1959.*

p. 160, footnote   Alex Comfort: "The Life Span of Animals," *Scientific American*, Vol. 205 (1961), p. 118.

p. 161, l. 18   Jack Kratchman and Douglas Grahn: *Relationships Between Geologic Environment and Mortality from Congenital Malformation*, TID–8204 (Washington: U. S. Atomic Energy Commission Technical Information Service; January 1960), p. 1.

p. 161, l. 32   Theodore T. Puck: "Radiation and the Human Cell," *Scientific American*, Vol. 202 (1960), p. 150. See also Theodore T. Puck: "*In Vitro* Studies on the Radiation Biology of Mammalian Cells," in *Progress in Biophysics, Vol. 10* (London: Pergamon Press; 1960), pp. 241-2, 255-6.

p. 166, l. 2   The National Advisory Committee on Radiation: *Report to the Surgeon General on the Control of Radiation Hazards in the United States*, U. S. Public Health Service (mimeographed; March 1959), p. 3.

p. 166, l. 35   For a detailed discussion of the Tricho episode, see Anthony C. Cipollaro and Marcus B. Einhorn: "The Use of X-Rays for the Treatment of Hypertrichosis Is Dangerous," *Journal of the American Medical Association,* Vol. 135 (1947), pp. 350-3.

p. 167, l. 21   Jack Schubert and Ralph Lapp: *Radiation: What It Is and How It Affects You,* p. 172.

p. 169, l. 22   Cf. ibid., p. 49.

p. 169, l. 34   For example, Russell Morgan, testimony, *Radiation Protection Criteria and Standards: Their Basis and Use, Hearings before the Special Subcommittee on Radiation, of the Joint Committee on Atomic Energy, Congress of the United States, 86th Congress, 2nd Session* (Washington: U. S. Government Printing Office; 1960), p. 267. Also W. Serber: "Indications and Hazards of Radiological Procedures in Pregnancy," *Journal of the Albert Einstein Medical Center,* Vol. 6 (1958), pp. 69-72.

p. 170, l. 3   Jack Schubert: "Fetal Irradiation in Relation to Cancer Deaths from Fallout and Natural Background Radioactivity," in *JCAE, 1959,* Vol. 2, p. 1660.

p. 170, l. 6   Ibid. Jack Schubert and Ralph Lapp: *Radiation: What It Is and How It Affects You,* p. 258.

p. 170, l. 19   Alice Stewart *et al.:* "A Survey of Childhood Malignancies," *British Medical Journal,* Vol. 1 (1958), pp. 1495-1508.

p. 170, l. 23   John M. Dennis: "Association of Irradiation with Neoplasia in Children and Adolescents," *Annals of Internal Medicine,* Vol. 44 (1956), p. 582.

p. 170, l. 28   C. Lenore Simpson and L. H. Hempelmann: "The Association of Tumors and Roentgen-Ray Treatment of the Thorax in Infancy," *Cancer,* Vol. 10 (1957), pp. 42-56. C. Lenore Simpson *et al.:* "Neoplasia in Children Treated with X-Rays in Infancy for Thymic Enlargement," *Radiology,* Vol. 64 (1955), pp. 840-5. C. Lenore Simpson: "Radiation-Induced Neoplasms in Man," in *Proceedings—Symposium on Fundamental Cancer Research,* Vol. 12 (1958), pp. 339-44. The reader's attention should be drawn to the interesting discussion that follows Simpson's paper in *Proceedings . . . ,* pp. 344-5.

p. 171, l. 6   Cf. L. H. Hempelmann: "Epidemiological Studies of Leukemia in Persons Exposed to Ionizing Radiation," *Cancer Research,* Vol. 20 (1960), pp. 20, 25.

p. 171, l. 20   George Crile, Jr.: "Carcinoma of the Thyroid in Children," *Annals of Surgery,* Vol. 150 (1959), p. 956. For a similar report based on experiences in The Johns Hopkins Hospital, see E. Hunter Wilson and Samuel P. Asper, Jr.: "The Role of X-Ray Therapy to the Neck Region in the Production of Thyroid Cancer in Young People," *A.M.A. Archives of Internal Medicine,* Vol. 105 (1960), pp. 244-51.

p. 172, l. 8   Cf. Jack Schubert and Ralph Lapp: *Radiation: What It Is and How It Affects You,* pp. 104-5, 163-7.

p. 172, footnote   British Medical Research Council: *The Hazards to Man of Nuclear and Allied Radiations* (London: Her Majesty's Stationery Office; June 1956), p. 16.

p. 173, l. 17   Consumers' Union: "Medical and Dental X-Rays," *Consumer Reports,* Vol. 26 (1961), pp. 493-501.

p. 174, l. 6   *The New York Times,* May 15, 1961.

p. 174, l. 33   The National Advisory Committee on Radiation: *Report to the Surgeon General on the Control of Radiation Hazards in the United States,* p. 1.

p. 176, l. 3   Barry Commoner: "The Hazard of Fallout—Nuclear Bomb Test Policy Should Be Decided by All," *Student Life,* Washington University, December 10, 1958, reproduced in *JCAE, 1959,* Vol. 3, pp. 2174-5.

p. 176, l. 11   Cf. W. F. Libby: "Radioactive Strontium Fallout," *Proceedings of the National Academy of Sciences of the United States,* Vol. 42, No. 6 (1956), pp. 380-1, 383.

p. 176, l. 22   Letter from Herbert P. Loper to Hon. Clinton P. Anderson, February 19, 1959, in *JCAE, 1959,* Vol. 3, p. 2537.

p. 176, l. 27   A. W. Brewer: "Evidence for a World Circulation Provided by the Measurement of Helium and Water Vapour Distributed in the Stratosphere," *Quarterly Journal of the Royal Meteorological Society,* Vol. 75 (1949), pp. 351-63. G. M. B. Dobson: "Origin and Distribution of the Polyatomic Molecules in the Atmosphere," *Proceedings of the Royal Society of London,* Series A, Vol. 236 (1956), pp. 187-93.

p. 177, l. 20   Special Subcommittee on Radiation of the Joint Committee on Atomic Energy: *Fallout from Nuclear Weapons Tests: Summary-Analysis of Hearings, May 5-8, 1959* (Washington: U. S. Government Printing Office; 1959), pp. 24-5. For data on other short-lived radio-isotopes, see: William R. Collins, Jr., *et al.:* "Fallout from 1957 and 1958 Nuclear Test Series," *Science,* Vol, 134 (1961), pp. 980-4.

p. 177, footnote   *JCAE, 1959,* Vol. 3, pp. 2540-1.

p. 178, l. 12   E. B. Lewis, statement, *JCAE, 1959,* Vol. 2, p. 1552. Also E. B. Lewis: "Thyroid Radiation Doses from Fallout," *Proceedings of the National Academy of Sciences of the United States,* Vol. 45 (1959), pp. 894-7.

p. 179, l. 10 U. S. Naval Radiological Defense Laboratory: "Statement," in *Selected Materials on Radiation Protection Criteria and Standards: Their Basis and Use*, p. 464.

p. 179, footnote Cf. Federal Radiation Council: *Background Material for the Development of Radiation Protection Standards, Staff Report No. 1* (Washington: U. S. Government Printing Office; May 13, 1960).

p. 180, l. 18 British Medical Research Council: *The Hazards to Man of Nuclear and Allied Radiations*, p. 68.

p. 180, l. 27 Cf. G. Failla: "Discussion," in *Selected Materials on Radiation Protection Criteria and Standards: Their Basis and Use*, pp. 209-11. According to Failla, the one-tenth rule adopted by the I.C.R.P. was not "intended" to apply to a "large population," although the terms "large population" were used in establishing the rule, and the rule was adopted by the A.E.C. Failla adds that there "has always been considerable reluctance on the part of radiation protection groups to make recommendations for the exposure of large populations: in the first place because of the limited knowledge concerning the effects of exposure at low levels of ionizing radiation; and secondly because the problem might well be considered to be outside the scope of their activities" (p. 210).

p. 181, l. 25 R. Björnerstedt and A. Engström: "Maximum Permissible Body Burden of Strontium-90," *Science*, Vol. 129 (1959), pp. 327-8.

p. 181, l. 35 W. O. Caster: "From Bomb to Man," in *Fallout*, edited by John M. Fowler (New York: Basic Books, Inc.; 1960), pp. 48-9.

p. 182, l. 24 J. Laurence Kulp *et al.*: "Strontium-90 in Man, IV," *Science*, Vol. 132 (1960), Table 5, p. 451.

p. 183, l. 7 Jack Schubert: "Additions to the Statement of Jack Schubert," in *JCAE, 1959*, Vol. 2, pp. 1641, 1643.

p. 183, l. 27 W. O. Caster: "From Bomb to Man," p. 49.

p. 184, l. 6 Paul Jacobs: "Clouds from Nevada: A Special Report on the AEC's Weapons Testing Program," *The Reporter*, May 16, 1957, p. 21.

p. 184, l. 23 Maurice B. Visscher: "Statement to the Subcommittee on Fallout Problems of the Joint Congressional Committee on Atomic Energy," in *JCAE, 1959*, Vol. 3, Table 1, p. 2142.

p. 184, footnote Cf. Edward Teller and Albert L. Latter: *Our Nuclear Future* (New York: Criterion Books; 1958), p. 94.

p. 185, l. 10 Cf. U. S. Public Health Service, tables on analyses of composite milk samples, in *JCAE, 1959*, Vol. 3, pp. 2178-87.

p. 185, l. 16   U. S. Atomic Energy Commission: "Results of Bread Analysis—New York City Samples," in *JCAE, 1959,* Vol. 2, p. 1257.

p. 185, l. 22   A. H. Sturtevant: "Effects of High Energy Radiation on the Human Body," in *Hubris, Man and Education, Papers Delivered at the Inauguration of James Louis Jarrett,* Western Washington College of Education (August 1959), p. 69.

p. 185, footnote   Federal Radiation Council: *Background Material for the Development of Radiation Protection Standards, Staff Report No. 2* (Washington: U. S. Government Printing Office; September 1961), p. 4.

p. 186, l. 6   James F. Crow: "Radiation and Future Generations," in *Fallout,* p. 105.

p. 186, l. 19   E. B. Lewis, testimony, *Hearings before the Special Subcommittee on Radiation of the Joint Committee on Atomic Energy, Congress of the United States, 85th Congress, 1st Session* (Washington: U. S. Government Printing Office; 1957), Part I, p. 962.

p. 186, l. 29   Cf. E. B. Lewis: "Leukemia and Ionizing Radiation," *Science,* Vol. 125 (1957), pp. 965-72.

p. 187, l. 6   Cf. Atomic Scientists Association: "Strontium Hazards," *Bulletin of the Atomic Scientists,* Vol. 13 (1957), pp. 202-3.

p. 187, l. 23   Ralph and Mildred Buchsbaum: *Basic Ecology,* p. 7.

p. 188, l. 18   U. S. Atomic Energy Commission: *Annual Report to Congress* (Washington: U. S. Government Printing Office; January 1960), p. 344.

p. 189, l. 1   Croswell Henderson *et al.:* "Effects of Low-Level Radioactivity in the Columbia River," *Public Health Reports,* Vol. 71 (1956), p. 13.

p. 189, l. 33   Lauren R. Donaldson: "Radiobiological Studies at the Eniwetok Test Site and Adjacent Areas of the Western Pacific," in *Biological Problems of Water Pollution,* p. 3.

p. 190, l. 16   L. R. Setter and A. S. Goldin: "Radioactive Fallout in Surface Waters," *Industrial and Engineering Chemistry,* Vol. 48 (1956), Table V, p. 254.

p. 190, footnote   Cf. Richard F. Foster: "Research and Development Programs Related to the Disposal of Reactor Effluent to the Columbia River," in *Industrial Radioactive Waste Disposal: Hearings before the Special Subcommittee on Radiation of the Joint Committee on Atomic Energy, Congress of the United States, 86th Congress, 1st Session* (Washington: U. S. Government Printing Office; 1959), Vol. 2, p. 1028.

p. 191, l. 6   Committee on the Effects of Atomic Radiation on Oceanography and Fisheries: *Radioactive Waste Disposal* *from Nuclear-Powered Ships* (Washington: National Academy of Sciences-National Research Council; 1959), Publication 658, p. 5.

p. 191, l. 15　K. Z. Morgan: "Summary and Evaluation of Environmental Factors That Must Be Considered in the Disposal of Radioactive Wastes," in *Industrial Radioactive Disposal*, Vol. 3, p. 2378.

p. 192, l. 26　Ibid. pp. 2389-91.

p. 194, l. 1　Walter Schneir: "The Atom's Poisonous Garbage," *The Reporter*, March 17, 1960, p. 22.

Chapter Seven:　Human Ecology

p. 196, footnote (l. 1)　J. B. Knook and R. D. O'Brien: "Effect of EPN on in Vivo Metabolism of Malathion by the Rat and Dog," *Agricultural and Food Chemistry*, Vol. 8 (1960), pp. 198-203.

p. 196, footnote (l. 8)　John W. Berg: "Looking at Cancer," *CA: Bulletin of Cancer Progress*, Vol. 11 (1961), p. 72.

p. 197, l. 2　James M. Hundley: "Statistics on Health," in *Food: The Yearbook of Agriculture, 1959*, pp. 177-8.

p. 197, l. 8　U. S. Department of Commerce: *Statistical Abstract of the United States, 1960* (Washington: U. S. Government Printing Office), Table 65, p. 60. See also Iago Galdston: *The Meaning of Social Medicine* (Cambridge, Mass.: Harvard University Press; 1954), pp. 82-3.

p. 198, footnote　U. S. Public Health Service: *Health Statistics from the U. S. National Health Survey, Selected Health Characteristics by Area, Series C-No. 5* (Washington: U. S. Government Printing Office; 1961), p. 1.

p. 199, l. 22　Alexis Carrel: *Man, the Unknown*, p. 111.

p. 202, l. 26　David Cort: "Reducing Ad Absurdum," *The Nation*, Vol. 192 (1960), p. 512.

p. 203, l. 17　Alexis Carrel: *Man, the Unknown*, p. 4.

p. 204, l. 18　A. F. Morgan and L. M. Odland: "The Nutriture of People," in *Food: The Yearbook of Agriculture, 1959*, p. 217. See also Agnes Fay Morgan (ed.): *Nutritional Status, U.S.A.*, Bulletin 769, California Agricultural Experiment Station, October 1959, pp. 40-77.

p. 204, l. 32　Alexis Carrel: *Man, the Unknown*, p. 112.

p. 205, l. 30　Cf. Roger J. Williams: *Biochemical Individuality* (New York: John Wiley & Sons, Inc.; 1956), p. 108.

p. 207, l. 8　Rene Dubos: *The Mirage of Health*, p. 155. Dubos's views seem to be based on the work on Anton J. Carlson and

Frederick Hoelzel: "Apparent Prolongation of the Life Span of Rats by Intermittent Fasting," pp. 363-75. See also "Nutrition, Health, and Longevity," *Nutrition Reviews,* Vol. 19 (1961), pp. 305-6.

p. 207, l. 27   Experimental work by Richard Eckstein, of Western Reserve University, summarized in *Highlights of Health Progress, 1956* (Washington: U. S. Government Printing Office), Public Health Service Publication No. 535, p. 2.

p. 207, l. 31   J. N. Morris and P. A. B. Raffle: "Coronary Heart Disease in Transport Workers—A Progress Report," *British Journal of Industrial Medicine,* Vol. 11 (1954), pp. 260-4. Special note should be taken of the table on p. 263 of this paper.

p. 207, l. 35   Hans Kraus *et al.:* "The Role of Exercise in the Prevention of Disease," *GP* (General Practitioner), Vol. 20 (1959), p. 121.

p. 208, l. 14   Rene Dubos: *The Mirage of Health,* pp. 155-6. For a brilliant discussion on caloric restriction and longevity, see C. M. McCay and Mary F. Crowell: "Prolonging the Life Span," *Scientific Monthly,* Vol. 39 (1934), pp. 405-14. See also "Nutrition, Health, and Longevity," *Nutrition Reviews,* Vol. 19 (1961), pp. 305-6.

p. 209, l. 8   George M. Briggs: "Unidentified Substances," in *Food: The Yearbook of Agriculture, 1959,* p. 349.

p. 211, l. 7   Edward Higbee: *The American Oasis* (New York: Alfred A. Knopf, Inc.; 1957), p. 161.

p. 212, l. 18   Ibid., p. 140.

p. 213, l. 14   Cf. U. S. Department of Commerce: *Statistical Abstract of the United States, 1960,* Table 925, p. 685.

p. 213, l. 23   Edward H. Graham: *Natural Principles of Land Use* (New York and London: Oxford University Press; 1944), pp. 153, 155.

p. 214, l. 8   William A. Albrecht, address before the Annual Meeting of the National Audubon Society, New York City, November 10, 1958.

p. 214, l. 16   George L. McNew: "The Effects of Soil Fertility," in *Plant Diseases: The Yearbook of Agriculture, 1953,* pp. 108, 114.

p. 214, l. 29   Claude Wakeland: *The High Plains Grasshopper,* U. S. Department of Agriculture (Washington: U. S. Government Printing Office; 1958), Technical Bulletin No. 1167, pp. 75, 99-108.

p. 215, l. 1   Edward H. Graham: *Natural Principles of Land Use,* p. 150.

p. 215, l. 6   Cf. Reginald Painter: *Insect Resistance in Crop*

Plants (New York: The Macmillan Company; 1951). C. P. Clausen: *Biological Control of Insects in the Continental United States,* U. S. Department of Agriculture (Washington: U. S. Government Printing Office; June 1956), Technical Bulletin No. 1139. James K. Holloway: "Weed Control by Insect," *Scientific American,* Vol. 197 (1957), pp. 56-62.

p. 216, l. 22   For a fascinating comparison between British and American agriculture, see A. N. Duckham: *American Agriculture—Its Background and Lessons,* Ministry of Agriculture and Fisheries (London: Her Majesty's Stationery Office; 1952).

p. 216, l. 31   Robert S. McGlothin: "Trends Within the Agricultural Industry," *SRI Journal* (Journal of the Stanford Research Institute), Third Quarter (1960), reproduced in *Current,* November 1960, pp. 45-6.

Chapter Eight: Health and Society

p. 220, l. 24   Iago Galdston: *The Meaning of Social Medicine,* pp. 31-2, 92.

p. 221, l. 35   John Shaw Billings: *Germs and Epidemics,* quoted in ibid., p. 44.

p. 223, l. 27   Rene Dubos: *The Mirage of Health,* p. 219.

p. 226, l. 22   Ibid., pp. 227-8.

p. 229, l. 18   Cf. Oscar E. Anderson, Jr.: *The Health of a Nation: Harvey W. Wiley and the Fight for Pure Food,* pp. 69-70, 77-80.

p. 230, l. 27   Letter to Robert Allen, June 4, 1906, quoted by Oscar E. Anderson, Jr.: *The Health of a Nation: Harvey W. Wiley and the Fight for Pure Food,* p. 188.

p. 230, l. 30   The role of Sinclair's novel in contributing to the passage of the pure food and drug law is vividly described in Robert B. Downs's afterword to *The Jungle* (New York: The New American Library of World Literature; 1960 printing), pp. 344-6.

p. 231, l. 15   Oscar E. Anderson, Jr.: *The Health of a Nation: Harvey W. Wiley and the Fight for Pure Food,* p. 203.

p. 231, l. 29   For a sympathetic presentation of Wiley's views, see Maurice Natenberg: *The Legacy of Doctor Wiley* (Chicago: Regent House; 1957).

p. 232, l. 10   Cf. Harvey W. Wiley: *The History of a Crime Against the Food Law* (Washington: Harvey W. Wiley, M.D., publisher; 1929).

p. 233, l. 9   Public Law 85-929, 72 *Stat.* 1786.

p. 233, l. 15   George P. Larrick, testimony, *Food Additives: Hearings before a Subcommittee of the Committee on Interstate and Foreign Commerce, House of Representatives, 85th Congress* (Washington: U. S. Government Printing Office; 1958), pp. 453-4.

p. 233, l. 24   Hon. James J. Delaney: "An Address before the National Health Federation" (mimeographed; 1958), p. 7; furnished by Congressman Delaney.

p. 234, l. 11   Arthur S. Flemming, testimony, *Color Additives*, p. 73.

p. 235, l. 4   For many natural alternatives to synthetic food additives, see the *Handbook of Food and Agriculture*, edited by Fred C. Blank. The book must be reviewed as a whole because no attempt is made to present these alternatives in a systematic fashion.

p. 235, l. 24   National Association of Frozen Food Packers, statement, *Food Additives*, pp. 408-9.

p. 236, l. 22   George A. W. Boehm: "The Noisome Problem of Car Fumes," *Fortune*, January 1960, p. 114.

National Cancer Institute, 141
National Committee on
  Radiation Protection, 174
  strontium-90, MPC, 180–81
National Health Federation,
  233
National League of Cities, xlix
National Resources Defense
  Council, lxvi
Natural Selection, affected by
  man, 60
Nature
  attitudes toward, 26, 52–53,
    240
  balance of, 29–30
  capitalism's effect on, xxxii
  environmental crisis and, lv
  exploitation of, 53
  and human ecology, 201–2
  and technology, 201–2
Naval Radiological Laboratory,
  U.S., 179
N.C.R.P., see National
  Committee on Radiation
  Protection
Nebraska, water-borne hepatitis
  in, 85
Nelson, Gaylord, xxxvi
Neoplasm, see Cancer
Nerve disorders
  from agene, 112
  MSG and, xxxviii
Netherlands, damage from
  emulsifier, 94
Neutron, 156
Nevada
  fallout in, 183–84
  underground nuclear tests in,
    liv
New Jersey, X-ray technicians
  certified in, lx
New Haven, Conn., lead
  exposure in, xxiii
New York City
  asbestos poisoning in, xxx
  during 1930s, li

solid waste disposal in, xlix–l
strontium-90 in milk and
  bread, 185
subway noise levels in, li
survey on radiation practices,
  174
New York City Cancer
  Committee, survey, 152
New York State
  radiation-induced mutations
    in, 160–61
  X-ray technicians certified in,
    lx
New York State Air Pollution
  Control Board, report,
    80
New York State Health
  Department, lead
  concentration study, xxv
New York Times, xiii, xx
New York-New Jersey
  metropolitan area, asbestos
  poisoning in, xxix
Niacin
  losses due to blanching, 92
  variation in sweet corn, 91
  See also Vitamin B
Nickel, xxiii
  as carcinogen, xxxi
Niobium, xxxi
Nippon Nitrogen (Chisso
  Corporation), xxv
Nitrates
  in meats, xliv, 115
Nitrites, xlix
  carbon monoxide and,
    synergistic effect, xvii
  in meats, xliv, 115
  toxicity of, 116
Nitrogen
  interaction with soil cations,
    45–46
  oxides of, 81–82
Nitrogen cycle, inorganic
  nitrogen fertilizers and,
    liii

Paint industry, xxiv
mercury compounds used by, xxvi
Paper industry, mercury compounds used by, xxvi
Parathion, 99
Paris green, 98
Pasteur, Louis, 222
Paul, Allen B., 89–90
PCBs, see Polychlorinated biphenyls
Pellagra, 20
Peller, Sigismund, xvi, 122–23, 136, 143
Pelvitmetries
and cancer in children, 170, 186–87
in England and U.S., 170
Pendergrass, Eugene P., 129, 131
Penicillin
allergies, 107–8
germ resistance to, 108–10
use as growth promoter, 106
Peptic ulcer, 70–71
Percy, Charles, xlvii
Pesticides, xiv
in agriculture, 97
cadmium poisoning and, xxviii
chlorinated hydrocarbons and as, xxi
production of, 103–4
residues, 98, 101, 103
See also Insecticides
Pests
and agricultural diversity, 213–14
biological control, 54
infestations from over-grazing, 214
and soil fertility, 214
Petroleum distillates, carcinogenic properties, 142
Pettenkofer, Max Von, 221–22

Pharmaceutical industry, xiii
mercury compounds used by, xxvi
Philadelphia *Evening Bulletin*, xxxvi
Phosphate detergents, xliv
Phosphate rock, lx
Physical activity
and health, xviii, 207, 219
during Renaissance, 63
Physiology
limited knowledge of, 203
and work, 63–64
Pittsburgh, air pollution in, 85–86
Plankton, concentration of radioactive wastes, 189–90
Plant nutrition, views on, 32–33, 45–46
Plants
lead poisoning and, xxiv
physiology of, 45–46
and soil maintenance, 34–35
Plastics, lii
polyvinyl chloride, xliv, xlv
Pleural calcification, asbestos poisoning and, in Finland, xxx
Plutonium-239
breeder reactor and, lxvi–lxvii
waste from Hanford installation, lxviii
Polio, water-borne, 85
Pollution, see Air pollution; Radioactive wastes; Smog; Water pollution
Polychlorinated biphenyls (PCBs), xxiv
contamination and effect of, xxii–xxiii
Polyoxyethylene derivatives
in processed foods, 116–17
toxicity of, 112–13
Polyoxyethylene (8) sterate, toxicity of, 112–13

74 75 76 77 10 9 8 7 6 5 4 3 2 1